EMBRACE EVERY MOMENT

Live Fully Live Now

BENEDICTA G. OLAGUNJU

Copyright © 2024 Benedicta G. Olagunju All rights reserved.

No part of this publication may be produced, distributed, or transmitted in any form or by any means, including photocopying, recording, or other electronic or mechanical methods, without the prior written permision of the publisher, except in the case of brief quotations embodied in critical reviews and certain other noncommercial uses permitted by copyright law.

For permission requests, write to the publisher, addressed "Attention: Permissions Coordinator" at the email address below:
Life and Success Media Ltd
e-mail: info@abookinsideyou.com
www.abookinsideyou.com

Unless otherwise stated, all scriptural references are taken from the King James Version of the Bible. Other versions cited are NIV, NKJV, AMP and KJV. Quotations marked NIV are taken from the HOLY BIBLE, NEW INTERNATIONAL VERSION.
Copyright © 1973, 1978, 1984 by International Bible Society. Used by permission of Hodder and Stoughton Ltd, a member of the Hodder Headline Plc Group. All rights reserved.
"NIV" is a registered trademark
of International Bible Society. UK trademark number 1448790.
Quotations marked KJV are from the Holy Bible, King James Version.

EMBRACE EVERY MOMENT
ISBN: 978-1-8380040-6-4

Cover Design: **MIA**DESIGN.COM

Contents

Foreword [9]

Chapter 1: Your Time Starts Now [15]

Chapter 2: How Long Is Life? [35]

Chapter 3: Made Through The Process [47]

Chapter 4: A-Z of a Successful Life on Earth [67]

Chapter 5: Jesus, The Answer; Lessons From The Healing of Blind Bartimaeus [105]

Chapter 6: Old Age - A Crown or A Thorn [127]

Chapter 7: Foes in Friends Cloak [145]

Chapter 8: I am Single, So What? [173]

Chapter 9: The Deceit of Youthfulness [187]

Chapter 10: The Ungrateful Thorn; Rising Above The Pain of Ingratitude [201]

Dedication

To my Heavenly Father, thank you for always standing by me during tough times. You have seen me pick up the pieces of my broken heart more than I can say. Thank you for teaching me what life is about and how to enjoy every moment.

To the people who have taught me valuable life lessons, your wisdom has made a big difference in my life. You have helped me pass on hope and encouragement to others, just like you did for me.

To everyone going through hard times, facing both good and bad moments, and maybe losing sight of what truly matters, I hope you find new hope and a fresh start. May you live fully and embrace every moment.

This book, EMBRACE EVERY MOMENT (Live Fully, Live Now), reminds us to make the most of our lives.

Acknowledgement

I want to express my profound appreciation to my Heavenly Father, who inspired me to write this book. His guidance is essential and paramount to me, and without His help, this journey would not have been possible.

I want to express my deep gratitude to my incredible husband and our three wonderful children, who are now adults, for their support and love. Your presence enriches my life in countless ways, and words cannot fully express my appreciation for everything you all do. Thank you for being my constant source of joy and inspiration.

Thank you to my family and friends for your continuous support. You have been there for me, cheering me on and encouraging me to keep moving forward. I am incredibly grateful for your love and belief in my vision.

Thank you to everyone who has been part of this journey. Your kindness and support have been a great encouragement to me.

This book is for anyone seeking direction and meaning in life. I hope it reminds you that you are not alone and that a fulfilling, joyful life is within reach. Therefore, I welcome you to join me as we each strive to embrace every moment of our lives with God's strength to live fully and live now.

Foreword

Imagine finding yourself on a narrow, winding path in a dense forest. Each step forward is an act of trust, a belief in the journey, even when the destination is not in sight. The path twists and turns, offering glimpses of sunlight through the canopy above, moments of clarity and warmth on your face. This path, with its unknowns and revelations, embodies the spirit of "Embrace Every Moment (Live Fully, Live Now)." It is not just a book but also a guide that invites you to slow down, notice, and live deliberately amid life's inevitable complexities, making it highly relevant to your growth's journey.

Life, in all its complexities, boils down to the simple moments we often overlook - the quiet mornings, the spontaneous laughter, the unexpected conversations that linger in our memory long after they are over, and many others. These are the actual fibres of joy and fulfilment. Yet, in our rush to meet expectations and milestones, we often glide past them, unaware of the richness they add to our lives.

Here, the author invites us to pull the emergency brake, not to halt our journey, but to slow down enough to see, feel, and truly experience our journey. Through each carefully crafted chapter, the author extends an invitation to read and engage deeply with the unfolding narrative of our own lives. From the awakening call in "Your Time Starts Now" to the pain of ingratitude in "The Ungrateful Thorn," each segment of this journey challenges us to pause, reflect, and ultimately transform. It is a call urging us not to settle for the status quo but to embrace change, growth, and the fullness of life. This is not about stopping our progress but enriching it, ensuring that by the time we turn the final page, we are not just revived and refreshed but also ready to flourish, fly, and fruitfully fertilise each day with the wisdom contained within these pages.

The journey through "Embrace Every Moment" is rich, inclusive, and universal. It offers something for everyone, whether young or old, single or married, or male or female, making it clear that growth, change, and fulfilment are accessible to all who embark on this journey.

As you embark on this path, each chapter becomes a stepping-stone in understanding and application, marking a journey of renewal and empowerment. Equipped with the tools to thrive in the business of living, this book serves as a veritable instrument in your toolkit for life, nurturing an ever-increasing potential to do more, to be more.

I highly recommend this incredible and inspiring book as your companion in discovering the richness of the present moment. So, live fully, live now, because this moment, right here, is life! Here is to the journey ahead. Happy reading!

Dr Joan Myers OBE
Founder, Joan Myers Consultancy Ltd.

INTRODUCTION

On a journey not too long ago, I reconnected with an old friend, and we started talking. We did a lot of catching up, and along the line, I asked about her life, and she became quiet and visibly shaken. I quickly said, "Sorry," thinking I had upset her.

Nevertheless, she reassured me, saying it was not my fault. Then, she shared her story. Life had been tough on her, filled with experiences—the good, the bad, and the downright ugly. These experiences had kept her from really living her life. At one point, she started going with the flow, waking up each day to do whatever came her way, whether or not it mattered to her.

EMBRACE EVERY MOMENT

Many of us are caught up in things that distract us from the life we are meant to live. The only way to break free from these distractions is to grab every moment, using wisdom and acting quickly. We must say no to distractions, understanding that a meaningful life comes from making the most of every moment.

Today, we are all moving so fast, trying to do so many things at once. It feels like we are racing against time, filling our days with tasks, both important and not. For all its benefits, social media has become a major distraction, especially for young people, keeping many from living their lives to the fullest.

Many people feel stuck because of life's ups and downs. Everyone is battling something – tough times, the hustle and bustle of everyday life, or the hurt from being let down. This can make us pause and question how we are living our lives.

While some rise above and make the most of every moment, others struggle.

Embrace Every Moment is not just a book but also a personal journey. Benedicta, the author, shares her wisdom, which she earned through years of guiding others, to light your path. The book is a collection of real and imagined stories that will motivate you to live more meaningfully and teach you how to navigate life.

This book is not just a piece of advice; it is like a friend walking beside you, helping you find your way. From Your Time Starts Now to The Ungrateful Thorn, every chapter peels away the layers of distraction, disillusionment, and disconnection that life piles upon us, revealing the core of what it means to truly live. You will learn about facing life's challenges, appreciating every moment, and finding true happiness and success.

Benedicta, with her deep well of wisdom, offers not just anecdotes but lifelines – practical wisdom and spiritual insights that guide you through life's maze. Whether it is the challenge of navigating through the illusion of youthfulness, the solace in singleness, or the wisdom to discern friends from foes, Embrace Every Moment equips you with the tools needed for a successful life on Earth.

As you turn the pages of Embrace Every Moment, let each word, story, and lesson wash over you like the first rain after a long drought. Let it renew, inspire, and set you on a path of discovery and fulfillment.

Chapter 1
Your Time Starts Now

"Life is a JOURNEY, not a DESTINATION"
– Ralph Waldo Emerson

Gazing at the ceiling, her eyes cruised in exasperation. Within a few seconds, her entire life played out before her like a movie. But whether or not the movie will have a happy ending is dependent on the benevolence of God to grant her a second chance.

As she lay vulnerably on the hospital bed with the scenes of her life still playing out in her mind, the only wish she had at that point was to be given another opportunity to rewrite her life's story.

Kathy, a beautiful and lavishly endowed middle-aged woman was born into a reputable family. Life started for her on an interesting note. Being born into affluence made her life the envy of her contemporaries.

Pretty Kathy, as her peers fondly called her, nurtured many dreams as a child. While growing up, one of her biggest dreams was to become a channel through which the downtrodden would find hope. Whenever she saw people living in abject poverty, it angered and awakened in her, a longing to become a helping hand to the poor. She would always jokingly tell her siblings that when she grows up, she would end poverty.

She always talked so passionately about how she would make the world a better place, prompting her peers to nickname her, "Poverty Alleviator." On many occasions, Kathy saw herself in a dream, pulling people out of the mud and helping them clean up. These constant encounters in her sleep world further solidified her conviction that she was truly born to be a helper.

Kathy continued to nurture her ambitions by always fantasising about how she would build a career after graduation, acquire wealth, and become a great philanthropist.

Soon, a series of events happened, which changed the trajectory of Kathy's journey. Upon graduation, she got married to her heartthrob. It was a memorable moment for her as she walked down the aisle with her dream man. The euphoria that came with being newly married overshadowed every other thing, including her biggest dream.

While Kathy was trying to settle in, pregnancy happened. Then, the realities of being married began to set in. As a result, she decided to pack up her dream of becoming a philanthropist until later years. Kathy made up her mind to focus on building her marriage and career, make loads of money, retire at 55, and venture fully into philanthropy, which to her, was the only thing that could give her complete fulfilment in life. However, the unimaginable happened.

Just a few weeks after her 52nd birthday, Kathy became critically ill. It was a devastating moment for her and her family. Would this discovery affect her plans of establishing her long-anticipated NGO to cater to the needs of the poor? Would she get a chance to make it alive, at least for the sake of the less privileged, for whom she had worked all her life, planning and saving up to cater to after retirement?

Kathy soon began to frequent the hospital every week for treatment. On this particular day, her entire life played out for her. As usual, she had gone to the hospital for a check-up. The doctor made her lie on the bed while he prepared the instruments needed for her check-up. As she lay down, she stared intently at the ceiling and got lost in deep thought recounting her journey so far.

The silence that enveloped the atmosphere was soon broken, as the doctor walked towards her bedside and gently whispered, "Madam, everything is ready for your check-up." Still lost in thought, she never uttered a word nor noticed the presence of the doctor.

"Ma'am," the doctor continued, "you seem lost in deep thought. Is anything the matter? We can talk about it if you don't mind." He patted her feet consolingly to make her feel at ease.

"Doctooor! Doctooor! Doctooor! Everything is the matter," Kathy muttered slowly, as tears began to well up in her eyes, with words choking in her throat while she struggled in between pain and tears pouring out her heart.

She continued, "It just dawned on me that I haven't truly lived. I have merely been existing, doing every other thing. I have birthed children, built a marriage and a profitable career while postponing the biggest dream that could have given me the greatest satisfaction and fulfilment in life."

"Doctooor! Doctooor! How I wish I had given attention to my biggest dream and built it alongside other facets of my life. But here I am, lying feebly on this bed, as this illness continues to spread, defying medical interventions. Here I am, not knowing if I will make it out of this ordeal. How I wish I could go back and truly live! How I wish I had EMBRACED EVERY MOMENT!

Just like Kathy, many of us have not understood what it truly means to live. Many, in a bid to build up empires for themselves and satisfy their fleshly desires, have paused their lives, postponing their dreams and purpose of existence.

Many have not yet come to terms with the fact that the day they were born was the day their lives started. Some think their lives would start when they graduate from school and secure a high-paying job or when they marry, build empires, have kids, and acquire some wealth. As a result, they shortchange themselves from truly living the lives they were created for. That was one of Kathy's mistakes.

As a way to bring this story home to help us evaluate our lives, let us consider a few mistakes that Kathy made that you can avoid today to ensure you do not end up in regrets as she did.

Mistake 1: There Was No Urgency Attached To Her Dream

It is one thing to have a big dream; it is another thing to understand the timing of that dream.

Kathy had a dream but did not feel a sense of urgency about it. She believed her dream was something that could always wait. From every indication, it was clear that alleviating poverty by extending a helping hand to the needy was a problem that she was designed to solve. It was her life's purpose. At least, her constant encounters with the downtrodden in her dream, and the irritation that she felt each time she saw people struggling to have the basic things of life, plus her regrets, proved so.

Kathy erroneously believed that she needed to acquire much wealth before attending to her dreams. That way, she would help people in bigger ways. She had a great vision, quite right, but missed out on the fulfilment that would have followed the attainment of that vision simply because she had no sense of urgency.

You see, it is okay to want to get things right before venturing into certain things, especially when it will require many resources. However, in trying to do that, you must not give in to complacency or become laid back in the pursuit of your vision. While trying to increase your mental, emotional, spiritual, material, or financial capacity for the vision, you must understand that timing is imperative. Hence, if you continue to wait to completely figure out your life before attending to your vision, you might later find yourself in a situation where, like Kathy, you have obtained all you want, acquired all the wealth, and are ready. Unfortunately, the vigor or opportunity to do it is no longer there.

Mistake 2: She Thought She Would Always Be in Control of Her Dream

Another mistake Kathy made was that in her planning, she did not factor the possibility of things going wrong or things not going according to her plans. This was one of the things that made her not feel any sense of urgency.

The truth is, whether or not you like it, things will not always go your way. Your health can fail you, just like Kathy's. In addition, death can happen and other misfortunes that you never anticipated can occur. No one plans to die, become ill, or be overtaken by misfortune. Sadly, this is life and life can happen to anyone at any time, whether they see it coming or not. You don't have to invite trouble for it to knock at your door. It can come unexpectedly. Kathy did not have to invite illness for it to strike. As I said, that is life for you!

It is also why, as a human, you must learn to be in tune with your Maker, as only He can make your plans succeed and avert any negativity the enemy may want to throw at you. Even the Holy Bible affirmed that for us to succeed in our plans, we need to hand it over to God, who has the power to establish it.

"Commit your actions to the Lord, and your plans will succeed" Proverbs 16:3 (NLT).

Mistake 3: She Did Not Figure Out Little Ways to Start Living Her Big Dream

Another big mistake Kathy made was that she felt things were within her control. She did not make an effort to figure out little ways she could start achieving her big dream.

"But what could she have done?" you might ask. Well, to answer that, Kathy could have started small without waiting until she was

55. Remember that this was a dream she started nurturing from her childhood. So, why wait until she was old before doing the major thing that could have made her life more meaningful?

She could have started by giving out personal stuff such as clothes, shoes, etc. that she no longer needed. Even as a teenager, she could do that because she

"If you cannot do great things,
do small things in a great way"
- Napoleon Hill.

came from a family of affluence. That also meant she did not live in lack. For her to always see people who lacked the basic things of life and felt bad about it meant she had something they did not have and wished to help them access those things.

Again, as a mother, she could cook during her birthday or children's birthdays and share with the needy people on the streets. She could also gather items that her children no longer needed to give to orphanage homes or even the poor children in her neighbourhood. She could cook and offer to beggars. During school resumption, as she was shopping for her children's school materials, she could add one or two extras to give out to any poor child she knew. Then, during Christmas, she could buy a few clothes for a less privileged kid. She could also help widows in her community. The list of what she could do to live her dream is endless. Interestingly, she did not even need millions to achieve all these.

Sadly, all she did was to fantasise about her vision, waiting to launch out big. I tell you, no matter what your dreams are or how gigantic they might be, there is always a small way to begin. As the saying goes, every big thing starts from little.

"If you cannot do great things, do small things in a great way" - Napoleon Hill.

Have you seen anyone who desires to build a house that started building it from the rooftop? It always starts from the foundation. Like the examples given above using the case of Kathy, you can apply the same method in building your dreams. You do not have to wait until you have it all figured out. Whatever lesson you are going to learn in your journey through any vision is engraved in the process. If Kathy had started with the little resources available to her, she would have learned how to grow big through the process.

As you read through the pages of this book, ensure it is not another opportunity to add to your 'bragging' list of how many books you have read. Rather, let it awaken in you a sense of urgency not to procrastinate on your vision and spur you into taking the right actions toward its attainment.

Little drops of water make an ocean. Hence, your little effort and actions in the right direction will go a long way to help you live a purposeful and meaningful life rather than just sitting and waiting to do big things that you might never do. Do not be like Kathy, who only fantasised but never did.

Let these words from Arthur Ashe guide you."Start where you are. Use what you have. Do what you can." As the Bible states, *"Do not despise the days of little beginning,"* many people despise what they have by constantly looking down on it or comparing it with what others have. By so doing, they end up not maximising their gifts. What you despise, you cannot maximise. You can always do something with what you have to get started in life. Waiting until it becomes bigger before you start is synonymous with wasting that which you have.

Some people think they can never truly start living their dreams until they have all their problems solved or everything properly figured out. But that is a lie they have allowed to cage them from truly living. Life is not something you pause to sort out other stuff and then come back to it. Life is meant to be lived and embraced every minute.

As Emerson asserted in the opening quote, life is a journey, not a destination, it has some questions for you.

Have you begun your journey through life? Have you started embracing every moment that life offers you? Take a moment to reflect on that.

Now that you have read Kathy's ordeal, what should you do to ensure that you do not end up in regrets as she did? I can tell you emphatically that the regrets of not trying surpass that of failing. The regret of knowing that you did not fully maximise

>
> "Start where you are. Use what you have.
> Do what you can."
> - Arthur Ashe

your life here on earth is too painful. Nevertheless, the great news is that you can evade it. Below is how to prevent regrets in life:

"Run As If You Stole Something."

Yes, you read that right. Run with your dreams like one who is being chased for stealing a valuable piece.

In the heart of the night, under the cloak of darkness, imagine the feeling of running as if you have stolen something. This is not merely about the adrenaline-fueled sprint of a thief fleeing a scene; it is about embracing the intensity, the urgency, and the unrestrained commitment to propel yourself forward, against all odds, towards your dreams and aspirations.

"Run like you stole something" is a powerful call-to-action to every dreamer, fighter, and soul yearning for a change. It is a summon to unleash the untapped reserves of strength and determination within you, to dash with the ferocity of someone with everything to lose yet everything to gain. It is about running with a heart so fierce, so driven, that the world around you becomes blurred, leaving nothing but the pounding of your heart, the rhythm of your breath, and the relentless echo of your feet against the earth.

This is your moment – the moment to chase your dreams with the intensity of a storm, to pursue your goals with the tenacity of a warrior, and to live your life with the passion of a heart that knows no bounds. Run as if you have liberated the most precious treasure because, in truth, you have—your untapped potential, unexplored talents, and unwritten future are great treasures to be liberated.

Let every step be a declaration of your courage, every breath a testament to your resolve, and every heartbeat a reminder of the fire within. Run not away from the challenges that life throws your way, but towards the life you have always imagined. Embrace the sweat, the tears, and the pain, for they are the harbingers of your triumph. "Run like you stole something" is not just a metaphor for the speed of your strides; it is a philosophy of life. It is about running with such conviction and purpose that you leave behind doubt, fear, mediocrity, and everything that can hinder your velocity.

EMBRACE EVERY MOMENT

It is about seizing every day as if it were your last, loving as though your heart knows no hurt, and pursuing your dreams with an urgency that belies the notion of the impossible. So, lace up your shoes, set your sights on the horizon, and run. Run as if you stole something. Run like the wind – untamed and free. Run towards your dreams, your future, and your destiny. In this relentless pursuit, you will discover the essence of your being and the strength to become who you were always meant to be.

Run with the velocity of one being chased by a lion.

If Kathy had embraced every moment and run with her dream with such velocity, she would not have any reason to live in regrets later in life.

Chapter 2
How Long Is Long Life?

"You will only be remembered for two things: the problems you solve or the ones you create."
- **Mike Murdock.**

How long is a long life? If you throw this question open, you will be greeted by numerous views.

To one, a long life could mean living a hundred years or more, regardless of how it is lived, as long as it is long in terms of the number of years. To another, it could simply mean having the beautiful things of life and being on earth long enough to enjoy them, even if it is not up to a hundred years.

You can see that what long life means to one is not what it means to another. But for you, my dear reader, how long is a long life to you? You see, questions like this can evoke deep thoughts and emotions. I can tell that this question has probably not crossed your mind before now. But this is one of the questions that you should at least pause to ask yourself occasionally, as it can help you reflect on your life and make amends where and when necessary.

While you reflect on the question, permit me to let you in on what I call a long life.

A long life is one that is lived within the confines of purpose, the number of years notwithstanding. Life is not measured by how long it is lived on earth but how well.

From Mike Murdock's quote above, we can see that in the end, you will only be remembered for the problems you caused or the ones you solved. What that quote simply means is that by the time you come to the end of your life on this side of eternity, no one will care how long you lived, what will matter most will be the things you did with your life while you were here. Did you live it as a blessing or a curse to your generation? This calls for a sober reflection. Before you go on reading, pause for a minute and ask yourself, "With the way I am currently living my life, if God decides to call me home today, would the people who knew me while I was here be bold to say that my life was a conduit of blessing or a curse?" Ponder!

This brings us again to another definition of long life. It is a life lived consciously serving the purposes of God and being a channel of upliftment to humanity.

Aside from that, let us move to the next thing I want to address in this chapter. It is a powerful prayer that Moses made in the book of Psalms, which goes thus:

"So teach us to number our days, that we may apply our hearts unto wisdom." Psalm 90:12 (KJV).

As I move on to dissect the above scripture to help you understand better how you can truly live so that you don't end up in regrets, I want to assure you that the purpose of this chapter is not to instill fear of death in you, but to awaken in you a desire to live more purposefully. Let me begin with the A part of that scripture.

"Teach Us to Number Our Days..."

In this particular verse, we see Moses making a crucial prayer. Anyone who truly desires to embrace every moment and make the most of their existence on earth must align with that prayer. This is not a prayer for those who only want their lives to be measured by the length of their stay on earth but by the eternal investments they made while they were here.

Our lives on earth are numbered. Way before your arrival, God already knew you would be here. Similarly, He knows how long you would be here. Beyond that, He did not just bring you here to roam aimlessly and return home. He made you for a specific purpose.

Thus, Moses asking God to *"teach us to number our days"* is the same as saying, *"God, help us to realise that we are not going to be here forever."*

Many people live in denial of this fact. They tactfully avoid every discussion that can lead them to ponder this. Such people only want to wake up each day and live their lives in whichever way they think will be profitable. Whether or not purposeful living is captured in their daily activities is none of their business. As long as they can make ends meet each day, they are fine.

But is this truly how to live? I guess you already know the answer.

Life was not designed for humans only to make ends meet. If that is all God intended during creation, what is the point of making humans in His image and after His likeness when animals that are not made in His image are well-fed and cared for by Him without them having to labour for it? God's intention in the creation of man was to have an extension of Himself on earth. Moreover, you cannot truly pride yourself as an extension of God if all you do every day is to merely make ends meet. That level is for people who are still at the survival level where all they care about is to cater to their bellies. If you must become an extension of God on earth, you must align yourself with His purpose for you and go out each day doing things that thrust you to attain that purpose. Doing this becomes easier when you understand that your journey through this earth is temporal. Your days are numbered.

"...That We May Apply Our Hearts Unto Wisdom."

Before I dissect this B part of that scripture, let us consider the word 'that' derived from "Teach us to number our days 'THAT' we may apply our hearts unto wisdom."

Connecting the A and B parts of Psalm 90:12 with 'that' connotes that in learning to number our days, we can truly become wise. In other words, wisdom is a byproduct of living with the consciousness of the brevity of life. Knowing that your days are numbered will help you live your life with wisdom.

The more you understand that your life on earth is not permanent and that you are just a sojourner passing through, the more your heart will grow in wisdom to confine yourself within the purpose of God. It is also the case when you understand that God gave you the life you live and you will stand before Him to account for how you used the life He gave you.

With this, you can see the reason some people live carelessly. Their hearts have not learned the way of wisdom because of their inability to truly capture in the eyes of their minds the fact that life on this side of eternity is brief.

Because of how crucial the few things I am about to say are, let me reassure you once again that the purpose of this chapter is never to instill fear of death in you but to awaken you to purposeful living.

As stated earlier, life is brief. But this does not mean you should not desire a long life in terms of longevity of years. After all, life can still be long in number and meaningful in content. God, in His word, asserts, *"With long life, I will satisfy him and show him my salvation." Psalm 91:16 (NIV).*

From the above scripture, you can see that longevity is what God intends for everyone; it will not be out of place if you desire it. However, you must define a long life through God's word. Does God want us to merely live for hundreds of years with zero investment in His eternal bank?

When a person dies at age 120, we would call it a celebration of life. But for anyone who dies in the prime of their youthfulness, we call it a painful exit. In the sight of God, if the latter lived their short life with an understanding of Psalm 90:12 and with godly wisdom, were able to serve the purposes of God before their exit, while the former lived their long life in sin and wasteful ventures, the latter lived a longer and a better life.

>
> "It's not the years in your life that counts, but the life in your years."
> - Abraham Lincoln

Don't get me wrong. Living a long life is a positive thing that can be achieved by investing in your health and fitness. Being alive allows you to serve God and work towards establishing His Kingdom on earth. However, it's important to remember that the quality of your life is just as important as its length. Abraham Lincoln once said, *"It's not the years in your life that count, but the life in your years."* So, make sure to live a life full of purpose, meaning, and joy.

Being a mother, wife, minister of the Gospel, and philanthropist, and having lived for almost six decades, I can boldly say that I understand the importance of a long life in attaining one's goals. Even at this age, I still intend and pray to be here for many more years.

However, one of the things that have helped me achieve my goals and impact my generation is that I live daily with the understanding that life is brief and that any day can be the last. It sounds scary to live this way, but it has also allowed me to keep my life in check and invest my time and energy in things that are truly important to my journey. Living with the understanding that any day can be the last has helped me to embrace each moment with enthusiasm, gratitude, and a readiness to chase my dreams.

Once again, as I bring this chapter to a wrap, let me remind you that life is brief. But by EMBRACING EVERY MOMENT, your life will be memorable.

EMBRACE EVERY MOMENT

Chapter 3
Made Through The Process

"For me, becoming isn't about arriving somewhere or achieving a certain aim. I see it instead as forward motion, a means of evolving, a way to reach continuously toward a better self. The journey doesn't end"
- **Michelle Obama.**

Life is a process. For anything significant to happen in or around you, you must be willing to follow through the process.

Nobody ever emerges. Not every great person you have seen or heard of suddenly appeared. A process led them to greatness and shaped them into who they are.

For anyone you know who has ever made something meaningful out of their life or has achieved outstanding results, remember, it was not an overnight success. It was a process, a journey that they embraced and that led them to their achievements.

If successful people should open up to you about their journey to success, you will see that engraved in their stories are many nights of sleeplessness, days of toiling, failures, ups and downs, rising and falling, and discouragement. Nevertheless, the only thing that finally stood them out from many others was their tenacity not to give up on the right process.

You see, God created the earth and structured it so that for certain things to happen, the right principles must be applied.

Let's take the birth of Jesus as a case study. God made the earth in a way that for a new life to be birthed, it must be incubated in the womb for a few months.

Since Jesus is the Son of God who is going to come with the mandate of a Messiah, His birth did not have to be an aftereffect of intercourse between a man and a woman. Instead, He had to be the direct product of the Power of the Holy Ghost.

In that case, what do you think was the best thing for God to do? He should have just spoken Jesus into existence. After all, it was not as though He did not have the power to do it. He is God and can do anything, anytime and anyhow He deems fit.

However, because God understands principles and processes, He took the time to get a virgin who would volunteer her womb for Jesus to be incubated. Even when the woman doubted her possibility of becoming pregnant without knowing a man, God still took the burden of sending an angel to explain things to her understanding, all in a bid to obey His laid-down principles of how life should be birthed.

If God had to embrace and follow the right process to achieve His aim on earth, despite having the power to do otherwise, do you think you can become anything significant or achieve any great feat outside the right process? It is an impossible task!

Note that the emphasis is on THE RIGHT PROCESS, not shortcuts or a quick-fix approach. You cannot embrace and maximise every moment while despising the process. If you must embrace and make the most of every day, you must also be willing to submit to the process and price that each day will demand from you.

Let us go back to Jesus as a case study.

After His birth, God could have just made him grow overnight, considering that the mission He came for was crucial. Yet, Jesus had to submit Himself to the right process of growth.

He grew just like every other child in His days. He subjected Himself to learning. In Luke chapter 2, we see how He went to the temple with His parents. He even stayed back after His parents had left. What was He doing? He was busy sitting with the council of elders at the temple, learning and asking questions.

Remember that He is the Son of God, and had the nature of God and of man. Hence, he could have just beckoned on the Father to reveal everything He needed to know. Even so, He did not do that. Rather, He embraced every moment he had to learn by following the right process of learning and growth.

The Bible even recorded times when Jesus would sneak away from His disciples and go to a secluded place to pray, fast, and commune with the Father.

He knew the mission He came for, and willingly and humbly submitted Himself to all the processes that would prepare Him for His assignment.

Again, if Jesus, the Son of the Living God, had to follow the right process in fulfilling His assignment, do you think you can despise your process and achieve anything meaningful?

For anything you desire to become, a process will lead you to it.

For any height you want to attain in business, career, family, education, spirituality, or life generally, there is a process and a price tag.

In addition, you cannot despise the PRICE and expect to win the PRIZE. It has never happened and will not begin with you. It is in EMBRACING the PRICE that you can WIN the PRIZE.

Life itself is designed in such a way that everything has a price tag.

Do you desire a blissful marriage? **There is a price tag to it.**

Do you desire to live a life of meaning and impact? **There is a price tag to it.**

Do you desire a deeper relationship with God? There **is a price tag to it.**

Do you desire an excellent result in your academics? **There is a price tag to it.**

Do you desire to be a sort-after entrepreneur?
There is a price tag to it.

Do you desire to stay fit and healthy?
There is a price tag to it.

A price is attached to every height you want to reach; you cannot cheat or negotiate your way out of it. In supermarkets, once a price tag has been placed on products, there is no negotiation.

Similarly, you cannot negotiate the price on your desire or bypass the payment through shortcuts and quick fixes. You must pay in full. There are times when God will send you help as a consolation to encourage you. However, that does not negate the role you have to play in the actualisation of your desire.

Your growth is embedded in the process. As a result, it is only in diligently embracing the process that you truly grow.

If you're wondering what this process entails, let me explain it in the following lines.

WHAT IS A PROCESS?

The process is a series of steps or actions taken to achieve a particular result or outcome. It includes the challenges you have to face, the decisions you have to make, the battles you have to fight, and the mountains you have to climb through to attain a desired expectation.

This is why many people, especially the younger generation, tend to look for shortcuts because 'the process of' achieving anything is always riddled with many unpleasant experiences. Moreover, it is in facing and overcoming every challenge that results are achieved.

The process, though littered with twists and turns, can be highly beneficial to anyone who summons the courage to stay through to the end. You stand to benefit a lot when you conform yourself to the process that God has laid out for your journey to destiny.

Let's consider some of the benefits of staying true to the process.

Transformation: As you dream and daily go out in pursuit of the dream, God desires that you will achieve them, especially when those dreams are in alignment with His plan for your life. He is a loving Father who would not want you to dream in vain. However, as much as He is concerned about you and would want you to achieve your dreams, He is more interested in who you become while pursuing your dreams.

That is why He puts you through the processes that allow you to experience life in its diversity by passing you through the fire of refinement. The more fire you are exposed to, the more refined you become; the more refined you become, the more transformed you are. Remember, it is that transformed version of you that can handle the criticism and backlashes accompanying success. In other words, the essence of the process is to prepare you for greatness.

"Every new level comes with a new devil."
- Unknown

The fire in the process is not there to burn you to death but to refine and equip you for the beaming future you are dreaming of. The top attracts many enemies. A saying goes, *"Every new level comes with a new devil."* This is why God is more interested in producing a transformed you, who can handle all the challenges attached to that level you aim.

God knows that the process is not a walk in the park but a long walk of vicissitudes. That is why He made provision for your survival long before you even started dreaming of becoming anything. *"When you go through deep waters, I will be with you. When you walk through rivers of difficulty, you will not drown. When you walk through the fire of oppression, you will not be burnt; the flames will not consume you"* - Isaiah 43:2 (NLT).

In the scripture above, you can see that God did not assure you and me of a hiccup-free walk to destiny. Instead, He assured us of His presence in whatever situation we might find ourselves. The fire is there for your refinement and transformation, not destruction.

Stamina: Before I proceed with this, let me first establish what stamina is.

According to the Merriam-Webster dictionary, Stamina is the bodily or mental capacity to sustain a prolonged stressful effort or activity.

Other dictionaries define it as the physical and mental strength that enables you to do something or carry out a difficult and tiring task for a long period without giving up.

In other words, it is the CONTINUING POWER, the STAYING ABILITY, and the ENDURING CAPABLENESS you gain when you pass through the furnace of refinement that enables you to rise above life's vicissitudes.

You can only gain this kind of endurance as you journey to your destiny.

Because of the stamina you gain in the process, you will discover that you can no longer be tossed about by every challenge. With the fire comes an inner power to face your mountains without fear and fight with everything in you until victory is accomplished.

Patience: An Italian proverb says, *"Patience is a flower that does not grow in everybody's garden."*

This explains that patience must be a rare and vital virtue. By submitting yourself to the process that your vision demands, you can cultivate this virtue.

> "Patience is a flower that does not grow in everybody's garden."
> - Italian Proverb

Impatience is one of the many reasons people give in to discouragement and end up not achieving their goals in life. Impatience is also one of the reasons many people, including young, old, educated, uneducated, single, and married have messed things up and have shortchanged themselves from reaping the reward of victory.

Impatience kills but the virtue of patience is life to those who have them. If you are still wondering whether your goals are worth the stress and effort you put into achieving them or you are currently at a crossroads of confusion and wondering whether the result will be worth all the pain you go through, I tell you today that it is worth it.

You learn patience as you go through the process. With this patience, you become even more equipped to surmount bigger mountains in the future.

Indeed, patience is a virtue that is needed for your journey through life.

Obedience: It is not a man's nature to willingly comply with orders. Except there is a force compelling him to do so, man will naturally want to break the rules.

We see that in the fall of man in Eden. Eve was just a naive woman who danced to the tunes of the serpent to see things for herself by eating the fruit.

Curiosity was one of the tools that the serpent used to deceive her. It aroused her curiosity to discover things for herself, and she fell for it.

We also see how curiosity plays out in people's day-to-day activities. Tell a child not to touch something; by the time you bat an eyelid, that child is already touching it. Why is it so? They want to discover why exactly you ordered them not to touch it.

Tell a teenager that sex destroys, and they will want to taste it to find out for themselves what it is about sex that destroys.

It is human nature to want to disobey. That is why, even as believers, the Bible encourages us to walk in the Spirit because only the Holy Spirit of God can compel the spirit of man to want to obey God's command.

Isn't it interesting that by simply submitting ourselves to the process God has laid out for our journey we get to learn obedience?

So, while you see the process as suffering, God sees it as a way of helping you develop obedience. Do you see why the furnace is a place of making? God refines and prepares His very best through the process of the furnace.

Even Jesus, the Son of the Living God, had to learn obedience by the suffering on the Cross. The Bible recorded of Him in the Book of Hebrews 5:8, *"Even though Jesus was God's Son, He learned obedience from the things He suffered" (NLT).*

If Jesus had to learn obedience through suffering, why do you think God is going to teach you the same thing by pampering you unnecessarily?

Empathy: There is something about going through a difficult experience that opens your heart to accommodate others and feel their pain.

For instance, during the coronavirus era, there was news about people dying in some countries. I noticed that most people around me never took the news seriously.

Some felt it was just another piece of news making rounds. Others felt it was okay, as long as it did not get to their domain.

But I noticed that the same people began to feel more concerned immediately schools, worship centers, offices, malls, and markets were locked down. The same people who never showed concern began to do so. Why? It was because they had also been directly affected.

Although they might not have been affected directly by the virus, because their means of livelihood had been affected by the outbreak of the virus, they automatically began to feel the pain the rest of the world, especially those directly affected by the virus, felt at that point.

Some prayed in their closet and in the open for God to end the epidemic that had hit the world.

Empathy is a great virtue every human who desires to go far in life should have. By giving yourself to follow through on the right process, you get to develop this virtue and other godly virtues that will make your life a wonder.

Dear reader, as I wrap up this chapter, let me remind you again that if you must EMBRACE EVERY MOMENT for a more meaningful life, you have to submit yourself to the process now because it is in the process that your character will be built.

Chapter 4
A-Z of A Sucessful Life on Earth

*"You define your own life.
Don't let other people write your script."*
- **Oprah Winfrey.**

In this chapter, I will show you how to properly define your life for a more successful and meaningful living, using the 26 letters of the English alphabets.

A - Affirmation: In my many years on earth, I have learned never to use negative self-talk on myself. I have discovered that whatever we consistently say to ourselves becomes our reality. Positive affirmation is one great way to motivate yourself and boost your self-confidence.

In life, you'll face situations that may cause you to doubt God and yourself. In these moments, intentionally remind yourself of God's Word by speaking it to your challenges and yourself. This is a proven way to succeed in life.

Note that I am not just talking about affirmations but POSITIVE AFFIRMATIONS. It is not about speaking; it is about the worthiness of what you are saying that truly counts because people can speak wrongly to themselves.

One great way to ensure you speak correctly and positively is to base your speaking on the scriptures. What has the

Bible said concerning you? Those should be the basis of your affirmations.

Dig deep into the scriptures, find out what the Word of God has said about you, affirm them, and continue to affirm them in your life and situation until they become your reality.

B - Believe in Yourself: Do you believe in yourself? Do you believe in whom God has made you? Do you believe in the gifts and potential God has deposited in you? Do you believe you are truly made in the image of God and after His likeness? Do you believe that things will always work out for you?

You become what you believe. Hence, what you believe about yourself is as important as the air you breathe.

Believing in yourself is not about being overconfident in yourself. It is not about becoming boastful or arrogantly proud.

Rather, it is about having a healthy dose of self-worth. It is about acknowledging and appreciating yourself as God's handiwork.

> *"Whatever we believe about ourselves and our ability comes true for us."*
> - Susan L Taylor

It is about recognising that the life you live is the breath of God and that He has put so much into creating you. As such, you cannot be less of who He has made you to be.

It is about believing in all the abundance and uniqueness that God has invested in you and deciding that as long as you have breath, all of His investment in you will be fully maximised to the glory of His name. In the words of Susan L Taylor, *"Whatever we believe about ourselves and our ability comes true for us."*

Nevertheless, can you believe in God's investments in you if you do not believe in Him as your Maker? It is easier to believe in a product when you believe in the manufacturer of the product. It is your belief (trust) in the integrity of the manufacturer that sponsors your belief in the product and its content.

"He who is not courageous enough to take risks will accomplish nothing in life."
- Muhammad Ali.

Similarly, folks struggle to believe in themselves because they do not believe in the integrity of the One who has created them.

C - Courage: No human has ever become or achieved anything significant outside of courage. Courage is an important weapon that individuals who yearn for greatness must have in their arsenal. *"He who is not courageous enough to take risks will accomplish nothing in life." - Muhammad Ali.*

David, seeing the enormous work before his son Solomon as the new king of Israel, admonished him in the Book of I Chronicles 28:20 *"David also said to Solomon his son, Be strong and courageous, and do the work. Do not be afraid or discouraged, for the LORD God, my God, is with you. He will not fail you or forsake you until all the work for the service of the temple of the LORD is finished"* NIV.

David had earlier planned to build the Lord a temple and had started putting things in place. However, being a man of war whose hands had shed much blood, God told him not to build Him a temple, and He (God) specifically told David that his son Solomon would be the one to build the temple because God had chosen him to succeed his father David as king of Israel.

As a result, we see David, from verse 11 of 1 Chronicles chapter 28, giving Solomon the plans for building the temple. In recognition of the enormous work that Solomon was to confront, his father charged him in verse 20 to never entertain discouragement.

David did not wish away the fact that there would be challenges along the way. He did not sugarcoat the throne as a place of merriment. Remember he was the outgoing king and as such, was familiar with the battles that the throne attracted. Hence, he did everything to ensure that he gave his son the requisite boost needed for the journey ahead.

In the next few minutes, follow me as we dissect the charge of David to his son Solomon.

There is a lot to learn from this, and I can tell you without mincing words that if you carefully read and apply this charge to your journey, there will be no limit to how far you can go in life.

Be Strong: David acknowledged the fact that the building of the temple would require a whole lot of strength. This includes spiritual, physical, mental, emotional, and economic strength.

If Solomon must succeed as King, he must be strong in every sense of the word.

The same thing also applies to you today; to succeed in any endeavour you must master the art of being strong. In the course of your journey to actualise your vision, you will encounter many things that will require your strength to overcome. Do not forget that this is not limited to physical strength alone. There are days that all you will need to scale through would be how strong you are mentally.

Courageous: being courageous means doing something that scares you. It's normal to have doubts, inadequacies, and fears because courage isn't the absence of these things. Yet, you can keep pressing against all odds.

David knew his son would be confronted with many obstacles as he set out to build the temple; hence, the charge for him to build courage.

And do the work: In this part of the charge, David reminded Solomon that his strength and courage must foster the work of God.

There is no point in building capacity if there is no work to invest it in. Your strength and bravery must be to help you fulfil your assignment.

Do not be afraid or discouraged: For David to have told his son not to be afraid or discouraged meant that he acknowledged that fears and discouragement would come, and it could come in any form or shape. But he should never give in to it.

You would think that since it was God who gave the vision or specifically chose Solomon for the assignment, it would be a smooth ride. But no, it doesn't work that way.

Challenges will come; even if God came to you face-to-face to hand over your life's assignment to you, it will still not exempt you from going through the difficult moments accompanying that assignment. So instead of wailing about the challenges, take David's advice to his son, personalise and internalise it until you are no longer afraid or discouraged. After all, God never promised us a life without troubles. He only promised to be with us in trouble.

For The LORD God, my God is with you: Having been through different phases of wars and seen how God came through for him even in his weakest moments, David assured his son of the faithfulness of his God to always be with him. He was not in doubt of the ever presence of God. He was certain that the same way God was with him all through his reign as King in Israel, He would be with his son.

Besides, it is only human to feel deserted sometimes. Amid your trouble, you might feel that God has abandoned you, especially when things keep getting worse despite all your prayers, fasting, and efforts. But if you take a moment to shut yourself out of all the noise around you, you will realise that God has been with you more than you know it.

To succeed in life, you need COURAGE.

D - Discerning: To be discerning means to be able to perceive things, understand things, or have a good judgment. It is the ability that a person has to differentiate between two or more things based on insight and proper understanding. This, in turn, enables them to make a better choice.

Discernment is something that every individual who desires to go far in life should long to have because it can help avoid getting into unnecessary trouble.

A person with a discerning heart sees beyond what is displayed and hears beyond what is said. With discernment, you can grasp and comprehend obscure things.

Although discernment involves using human reasoning and observation to measure words and behaviour, if you are a believer, the Holy Spirit can help you attain higher levels of discernment.

Some things can never be seen with the physical eyes or grasped by human reasoning except God reveals them to you. Discernment is a gift obtained because of having a deeper walk and relationship with the Holy Spirit.

Benefits of Discernment

• **It Gives Direction:** "Whether you turn to the right or to the left, your ears will hear a voice behind you, saying, this is the way; walk in it" - Isaiah 30:21 (NIV).

The kind of hearing described in the above scripture is not the one we hear with our physical ears. You need to be in tune with the Spirit of God to have such ears. Only those who have established a working relationship with the Holy Spirit can hear and recognise His voice. Jesus, in the A part of the book of John 10:27, affirms, "My sheep hear my voice." Only those who are His, not in lip service, can hear His gentle voice and recognise it.

Imagine the assurance coming from knowing that God is always with you to direct you on what to do and which way to go. What a privilege it is to know that you have His backing! With discernment, you will not have to wander aimlessly in confusion because, at every point, the Holy Spirit is there to guide you.

- **It Saves You From Error and Trouble:** Many people today fight needless battles simply because they lack discernment.

Have you ever been in a certain place and suddenly, began to feel uneasy and a need to leave that environment? Then, you looked around to ascertain if there is a reason you felt that nudge but could not find any. Yet, in obedience, you decided to listen to that still, small voice and left, only to hear later that something disastrous happened not too long after you left. The Holy Spirit can do that when we build an intimate fellowship with Him. He will train your heart and awaken your spiritual ears and eyes to discern obscure things.

- **It Helps With Decision Making:** Have you ever found yourself in a situation where you have to choose between two nearly similar options? You know that being in such a situation can be very hard.

However, with discernment, you will not have to be confused, at least not for too long. Whether in your choice of whom to marry, what business to venture into, what career to pursue, which country or city to base in, or which university to apply to, with the help of the Holy Spirit, who comes through discernment as you continue to deepen your fellowship with Him, you don't have to be perturbed.

E -Empathy: I talked about this briefly in the previous chapter but in this chapter, I want to consider how we can build empathy and how it can impact our journey through life to ensure success.

Do not forget that empathy is your ability to feel the suffering of others and understand their emotions by putting yourself in their shoes. It enables you to imagine yourself in the situation of other people, feel their emotions, and understand their perspective or opinion, which in turn helps you act compassionately toward them. The truth is, as you climb through the ladder of success, you need empathy. Empathy improves your relationship with others, and as you already know, you need human relationships to attain greater heights in life.

How to Build Empathy

- Pause and think beyond yourself.

- Listen to understand.

- Be kind with words; avoid derogatory words.

- Do away with "it can never be me" mentality

- Respect boundaries; know when your opinion is needed and when it is not.

F - Forgiving: In your journey through life, people will hurt you, and say nasty things to you. The more painful aspect is that some will not even think or realise that they have hurt you, while some will claim right, even when they are aware that they have done you wrong. Whereas some will take the good step to apologise, others will not give a hoot.

In whichever way, if you truly desire to go far in life, it behoves you to forgive both those who asked for it and those who did not and may never ask.

You are not forgiving them because they deserve it; you are doing so because you need your mental and emotional well-being intact for the journey ahead.

G - **Giving:** "Life's persistent and most urgent question is, what are you doing for others?" - Martin Luther King JR.

In a world brimming with greed and selfishness, heaven squeals with delight when any of God's creatures rows against the tide to live a selfless life.

As you go through life, you will face situations that will require you to look beyond yourself. At such points, your ability to put your needs aside to solve other people's crucial needs will determine, to a large extent, the level of impact you will make.

Life is not always about what you can get; sometimes, it is about what you can give. Giving is an important virtue that anyone who truly desires a successful sojourn on this side of eternity must possess.

H - Holiness: Holiness is a demand for anyone or any believer who wants to fulfil their purpose in Christ. Holiness is not an option; it is what God and destiny demand of everyone. Unless you uphold it, there are dimensions in God and heights you can never attain.

Purity in every sense of it is what is expected of you. You destroy your destiny when you indulge in sin - sin is a killer of destiny. Therefore, you must watch how you live your life.

You cannot live in sin and expect your life to produce godly results. Sin is a disconnector. Hence, when you begin to make it your companion, you will be disconnected from your Source (Christ). *"I am the Vine; you are the branches. If you remain in Me and I in* you, you will bear much fruit; apart from Me, you can do nothing"- John 15:15 (NIV).

> "Give up the struggle and fight; relax in the omnipotence of the Lord Jesus; look up into His lovely face, and as you behold Him, He will transform you into His likeness. You do the beholding - He does the transforming. There is no shortcut to holiness."
> - Alon Redpath.

One of the ways to attain a life of holiness and total submissiveness to God is to fix your gaze on Him. *"But we all, with unveiled faces, beholding as in a mirror the glory of the Lord, are transformed into the same image from glory to glory, just as by the Spirit of the Lord"* - 2 Corinthians 3:18 (NKJV).

Trying to live a holy life without making Jesus your focus will always end in futility. In beholding His face daily through the lens of prayer and the Word, we are transformed into his nature.

As Alon Redpath affirmed, *"Give up the struggle and fight; relax in the omnipotence of the Lord Jesus; look up into His lovely face, and as you behold Him, He will transform you into His likeness. You do the beholding - He does the transforming. There is no shortcut to holiness."*

I - Integrity: In life, you will meet situations where your integrity will be tried. You must stand your ground and do what is right, regardless of whose ox is gored. That will determine how well you will turn out in life.

Scores of people have slaughtered their destinies on the altar of bribery, corruption, and lies. They think they are wiser than those who stay through on the right process simply because of the immediate gratification their dishonesty attracts, not knowing that they are doing themselves more harm than good.

Honesty, truth, and integrity still pay, no matter how hard the world tries to water them down.

J - Justice: In a world full of injustices, finding someone who would choose to do what is right, not minding who is involved, is delightful.

There are so many injustices going on in the world today. Humans are killing their fellow humans; ritual killing has been on the increase in recent times. Internet fraud (yahoo-yahoo) is increasing daily because many young people no longer want to work hard. In all, everyone is looking for shortcuts to wealth.

More women are giving in to the pressure of the day, resulting to increased prostitution. Snatching of people's spouses no longer means anything to some. They can even live together comfortably without any sense of shame or remorse. Some families no longer care about the widows. They treat them like pieces of trash and go as far as denying them access to the properties they worked hard with their late husbands to acquire.

Many do not give a hoot about what happens to the poor, orphans, and the less privileged around them. The government can introduce any policy without caring how it affects the poor masses. As long as the leaders' selfish desires are achieved, they are okay. This is worrisome!

Dear reader, the world has never needed just men and women who will stand and insist until the right thing is done, as it needs it now. Would you be that one person who will stand for righteousness and justice, even if it means standing alone? Think about it.

K - Knowledge: There is a saying that the day you stop learning, you start dying. This is so true. In life, there will be times when you will come head-on with challenges and it is only your knowledge that can bail you out.

Note that knowledge is not only about going to school to acquire more certificates, even though that is essential too. All the same, I am talking about investing in your personal development.

Knowledge is not just a necessity; it is a powerful tool that you need in various situations.

Knowledge is light.

Knowledge is a sustainer.

Knowledge is a guard.

Knowledge is something to strive for if you truly desire to make headway in life.

Please permit me to ask how much time, energy, and resources you invest in learning.

You can learn new skills, read books, or enroll in classes on personal development. No knowledge, they say, is a waste. Even if you don't need the knowledge today, you can acquire them for future purposes. For instance, as a single man or woman, you can attend seminars or enrol in classes on marriage. Although you have yet to marry, acquiring the skills needed and learning in advance can help you prepare for marriage. It can also help you look forward to it and walk into it with the right mindset.

L - Love: Love is the greatest Commandment of God. No matter what you do for humanity, if your intention is not hinged on love, you have only wasted your time.

Love is crucial in our journey through life. Love is a universal language. There is no human, who cannot understand the language of love.

As you sojourn through life, you will encounter many people you think do not deserve love, but God expects you to love them regardless.

Every other thing I have or will talk about in this chapter finds its root in love.

Love will make you empathetic towards others. Love will make you eschew injustice. Love will make you always want to pursue peace at all costs. Love is a great virtue that you must contend for.

For that, love others genuinely, no matter who they are. No matter what they have or do not have, let your love for them not be based on their social status, political position, economic power, etc. Rather, let it be because they are your fellow humans and deserve to be loved.

As you genuinely love others, make yourself loveable.

M - Moderate: It is said that too much of everything is bad. This is true. If you desire to live meaningfully and responsibly, you must learn to do things in moderation - avoid extremes.

Many people suffer today because they do not know how to do certain things in moderation. Many have eaten and drunk themselves to the grave and some into illnesses that have incapacitated them simply because they disregarded the instruction to do things in moderation. It is wisdom to live a moderate lifestyle.

N - Noble: A noble life is not attained in rascality. To be noble is to show good personal qualities and high moral principles. That means you don't just wake up to do anything that presents itself. You weigh your thoughts to ensure they align with what is right. You also weigh your words against your values before you say them. Finally, you weigh actions on the scale of your moral principles before you react or act in a certain way. A noble lifestyle is needed as you aspire to success.

O - Optimistic: To be optimistic means to always expect the best and believe that things will turn out well regardless of the current situation. Sometimes, your optimism is all you need to scale through.

Always believe that things will work out for your good and that even when bad things happen, God in His infiniteness will still make it to work for your good.

The Bible counsels, *"All things work together for good to those who love God, to those who are called according to His purpose" (Romans 8:28).*

P-Peace: I got to a point in my life where peace became my strategy and way of life. Although always speaking the language of peace often made me appear foolish and weak, choosing it has always helped my relationship with God and others. It also improves my mental and emotional well-being.

In life, people will step on your toes and say nasty things to you and about you. Often, they do it knowingly to get on your nerves, and in most cases, fighting back may look like the most suitable thing to do. I have learned by experience that going the way of peace, although hard, is the best way to handle such situations.

This does not mean that you should open yourself up for attacks. It means you should surprise people by responding peacefully when they expect you to join them to fight dirty - not all fights are worth it, and you can still fight back with peace.

Q - Question: The skill of questioning is paramount as you travel to the land of success. When you don't understand something, ask questions. When you are confused, ask questions. When you don't know, accept that you don't know, and ask questions.

Don't think that you know everything. The moment you begin to think that you know everything, that is the first sign that you don't know anything.

"He who asks a question is a fool for five minutes, but he who does not ask a question remains a fool forever" - Chinese Proverb.

R - Reliability: I can write a whole book on reliability.

In a world where social media has become a place where everyone is trying to create content and be the first to break news to get likes and comments, it is becoming harder for people to be reliable.

Can people confide in you about their ordeal and trust that you will not make them a topic of discussion? Can people do business with you and be rest assured that you would keep your end of the bargain? Can God trust you with assignments and His burden for this generation, knowing you will not disappoint Him?

When people know that they can always trust you, it opens you up for recommendations and increases your possibility of succeeding in life.

S - Sobriety: In March 2024, I was told of a young man, nicknamed Orile, in Lagos, Nigeria, who took Ice (a hard drug popularly known as Colos), ran into a canal, and drank himself to death. The drug intoxicated him to the point of losing mental stability and thoughtfulness. Sadly, that led to his untimely death. He lacked sobriety, and it cost him his life.

Sobriety is the state of not being intoxicated by alcohol or drug. It is also a state of thoughtfulness and seriousness, which enables you to think clearly and live a moderate life. Sobriety is a state you should strive to attain if you truly desire to go far in life. You can never achieve or become much by always being intoxicated, unthoughtful, and unserious.

T-Tolerance: It is known that people will not always do what you want or behave as you expect them to. We are all humans, and can revel or make mistakes occasionally. When such happens, your ability to tolerate others will keep you from reacting negatively.

It takes patience and self-control to tolerate people. Let's face the truth; it is not an easy thing to do. However, in doing so, you can coexist with people and build destiny relationships that can aid you in the future.

U - Understanding: Always seek to understand before you speak or react/respond to an issue. Many people are so rash with words and quick to act that they often get themselves into trouble.

When people come to you with a complaint or situation requiring your input, wait to listen before proposing a solution. Listen to understand the situation. Properly understanding the situation will help you propose a valuable solution.

V - Vision: Vision is the image of yourself that you can see through the eyes of your mind. It is a picture you hold about your future; it is what you intend to become or achieve.

Without vision, you will roam on the road of life. Vision is a compass to those who have it. It gives direction and helps you know the activities that deserve your time, energy, and resources and which do not.

W - WISDOM: Wisdom is so vital that even the Bible calls it the principal thing. It then, beckons on anyone who lacks wisdom to ask God for it and it will be freely given to them.

There are twists and turns in life that only wisdom can help you navigate.

If you have all the other attributes discussed in this chapter but despise wisdom, you will still be grounded in life.

The Bible says that with wisdom, a house is built. House in this context does not only refer to physical edifice but also anything that can be built.

It takes wisdom to build a home.

It takes wisdom to build a business.

It takes wisdom to build a ministry.

It takes wisdom to build a life.

It takes wisdom to build a career.

It takes wisdom to build people.

It takes wisdom to build anything at all.

Wisdom is a principal thing and is life to those who have it.

X - X-Factor: If you must succeed in any area of your life, you must learn to pay attention to your X-factor.

Your X-factor is that thing that makes you unique. It represents those qualities, attitudes, and ways of doing things that people find unique and interesting about you.

It does not have to be big things. It can be as little as your smile. Whatever it is, find and value it.

Y - Yielded: There is a purpose for which you have been created. God did not just create you to live and die without making any mark or leaving your footprint on the sand of life.

God has a plan for your life and it behoves you to find out what this plan is and yield to it completely.

Many are struggling today, not because they are not working hard or making enough effort, but because they are labouring outside of God's plan.

Note that this does not mean that anytime you struggle with something, you are automatically out of God's plan for you. It does not also mean that being in God's plan will negate the place of challenges. Many people today are making their lives more difficult because they have refused to yield to God and His plans.

Z - Zestful: The Bible says that whatever your hands find to do, do it with all your might. Ecclesiastics 9:10.

Most times, it is not about what you do, but how you do it and the enthusiasm and passion you invest into it, that truly matters. How enthusiastic and passionate are you?

EMBRACE EVERY MOMENT

Chapter 5

Jesus, The Answer:
12 Lessons From The Healing of Blind Bartimaeus

"Healing is a journey. Each step is unique."
- Jennifer L Betts.

The story of Blind Bartimaeus is one Bible story that greatly interests me.

In the book of Mark, chapter 10:46-52, we see a man who has earned a name by his condition.

Imagine when you have gone through a particular challenge for a long time that people have come to know you and address you by your suffering. That was how long this man had suffered.

Although the Bible does not tell us whether he was born blind or whether he became blind later in life, for this man to have been nicknamed for his blindness tells us that he must have been blind for most of his life.

Nonetheless, we also see in the story how he went against all odds to encounter Jesus, the Mighty healer.

As I studied this scripture and meditated upon it, God opened my eyes to some lessons that we can glean from the life of Bartimaeus, which can also help us through our journey on earth.

Join me as I give you a life-changing ride through the 12 lessons I have carved out from the healing ofBlind Bartimaeus.

Lesson 1: He Acknowledged His Need.

Although it was not expressly written in the story that he acknowledged his problem, all his actions from the moment he heard that Jesus was passing to the point of his healing proved that he did not sugarcoat his condition or live in denial of his current state.

He was a beggar, who daily went out to sit by the roadside begging because that was the only thing he could do to earn a living. He recognised that he was just a poor beggar who needed something beyond alms from Jesus. He acknowledged his need. That simple acknowledgment influenced his actions, leading to his healing.

Many people today have not yet come to terms with the fact that they have a need and need help. Hence, they try to come up with many excuses to cover up. This refusal to acknowledge our lack and the need for help is why many people live fake lives to conceal their pain.

If Bartimaeus had lived in denial of his need or tried to pretend that everything was cool, he would have only heard that Jesus passed by but would never have tasted of His healing power. The healing of Bartimaeus is hugely predicated on the fact that he acknowledged his problem. Therefore, he cried out to the one he believed would solve it.

I do not know the issues in your life that you have been concealing with smiles, pretence, and fake lifestyle, trying to sell the lies that everything is okay. Meanwhile, you know that it is not and you need help.

I am not in any way suggesting that you begin to dress or look like your condition. This is far from it. But a simple acknowledgment that the challenge exists and that you need help can be all you need to triumph.

Hello, why are you still holding onto that broken relationship, refusing to accept that it is over and that the person may never come back? Why are you refusing to see things as they are? Why are you living in denial and hurting yourself the more? You will never find healing unless you come to terms with the situation, see things as they are, and begin to make peace with it. Your healing is on the other side of acknowledging the situation - seeing it for what it is and reaching out for help.

That was what Bartimaeus did. Remember that people had been giving him alms for years. However, the alms never solved his problem. But when he heard that Jesus was passing by, he knew the solution to his problem was at hand. As an intelligent man, he seized the opportunity.

To date, Jesus has not stopped passing by. It is up to you to tell yourself the truth by accepting that you have a need that only He has the answer to.

Lesson 2: he believed.

The story has it that as Jesus was passing by, a large crowd followed Him. They passed by the road where Bartimaeus sat and begged. Perhaps, there must have been a loud noise from the crowd, which made him enquire what was happening since he could not see things for himself. Hearing that it was Jesus passing, he screamed and cried to Him.

Do not forget that this man was blind, meaning he had never seen Jesus perform miracles before. I guess he had heard of it but had never seen it with his physical eyes.

Yet, he believed on Him based on what he had heard about Him. His actions from the time he heard that Jesus was passing by to the point of his healing also proved that he truly believed in the healing power of Christ.

You see, there are certain things we will never experience and miracles we will never taste until we start believing. Many people, like Thomas, want to see before they can believe. Believing because you have seen is faith, but believing even when your eyes have not seen is the bigger faith.

The fact that no graduate or millionaire has ever come out of your lineage does not mean God cannot achieve such with you.

The fact that everyone in your family had a broken marriage does not mean you cannot have a blissful and lasting marriage. God can begin a new story of successful marriages with you.

Many people today have defined themselves by their experiences and background. They have been so used to seeing people around them fail that they now believe they are destined to fail. But here was a man who had never seen the miracles of Jesus, yet he believed based on what he had heard of Him. He believed that Jesus could heal him, and Jesus, just as it is with His nature, did not disappoint.

What have you believed God for? What are those things that God has told you He would do? I encourage you today to hold on to His words, not minding what is happening in or around you. Believe Him, He will do it.

Lesson 3: He Acknowledged Jesus.

Upon hearing that Jesus was passing by, Blind Bartimaeus immediately began to cry out to him for help and mercy. He acknowledged Jesus as the Son of David, the merciful God with the power to deliver.

He acknowledged his problem as a blind, poor beggar. But away from that, he acknowledged that his problem was not beyond Jesus - if there is a problem to solve, there is Jesus to solve it.

Blind Bartimaeus did not call Jesus to remind Him of his condition. Instead, he called out to Jesus and went straight to ask for mercy, which he needed. He needed Jesus to look upon him with compassion. He was not in for stories and did not waste time because he knew that Jesus had the solution to his problems. With that understanding, he asked for help.

What about you and me? We are often so engrossed in our problems that we begin to think they are bigger than God.

The truth is, no problem, no matter how big or devastating it is, can ever be greater than God. God is Almighty.

Lesson 4: He Did Not Listen To Naysayers.

In verse 48 of that same scripture, you can see how people tried to shut Blind Bartimaeus up. They rebuked him, telling him to be quiet.

The truth is, as you journey through life, you will come across people who will try to discourage you. At such times, your ability to withstand the pressure from the crowd without letting it affect your resolve will determine how far you can go.

When the stone of discouragement is thrown at you, you can decide whether to be buried by it or use it as bricks to build a meaningful life. You can either allow discouragements from the crowd to weigh you down or thrust you forward to a better future.

Lesson 5: He Kept Pressing On.

As the crowd tried to quiet him, rather than give in to their rebuke, Blind Bartimaeus screamed even more and cried louder to Jesus. The more they tried to shut him up, the louder he cried to Jesus.

Because he knew that Jesus was the answer to his problem, he refused to be silenced by the rebuke from the crowd. I hope you know it was not just one person that rebuked him. Imagine how you feel when you want to embark on a journey of pursuing a valuable vision. Suddenly, the people around you, perhaps friends and families, who you expected to back you up, begin to discourage you by telling you how foolish it is to embark on such journey.

Now, compare that feeling to when a crowd is trying to discourage you. That was the kind of situation this man experienced. Yet, he did not allow it to stop him.

Sometimes, your victory will not depend on how long you fast and pray or on the strategies you know or apply, but on your ability to keep going regardless of the discouraging situations around you.

Lesson 6: Jesus Stopped For Him.

Because Bartimaeus did not stop calling out to Jesus for help, because he persisted and did not allow the crowd to discourage him, Jesus stopped and called for him to come. Oh, what a merciful Jesus! Blind Bartimaeus did not stop because he needed Jesus. However, Jesus, on seeing his resilience, stopped for him.

This tells you that no one is beyond the mercy of God. If Jesus can stop and reach out to a poor, blind beggar like Bartimaeus, He can also reach out to you. You are not too far that His mercy cannot find you.

Dear reader, what are you going through that makes you feel abandoned?

What is that sin you are struggling with that has made you feel God cannot forgive you?

I tell you today that the mercy of God is available for you. Jesus loves you and desires to help and deliver you. Nevertheless, all He wants is to see a willing heart.

Blind Bartimaeus got Jesus' attention because he acknowledged his need for Jesus and showed a willingness to be helped.

Despite the crowd that followed Jesus, amid all the noise from the crowd, He still heard the cry of this poor man and reached out to him. Who told you that your prayers are not being heard? Who told you that because Jesus did not respond the first time you called, it automatically means He will never respond? Keep praying; your answers will come.

Lesson 7: His Naysayers Became His Announcers.

When Jesus called out to the man, the people who tried to discourage him earlier announced that Jesus was calling him. They even encouraged him to cheer up and rise to meet Jesus.

Remember, it was the same crowd. The question that kept bugging me was, *"What made the crowd change words and attitudes towards the man? Did they suddenly become changed people?"*

The truth is, nothing changed among the crowd. It was still the same people. However, what made their language and attitude toward the poor man change was that they were humbled by Jesus' action. They might have thought that Bartimaeus could never attract the attention of Jesus.

In their mind, how could Jesus bypass all the 'worthy' people to reach down to a beggar? They must have learnt that day that everybody matters to Jesus.

However, if this man had listened to them earlier and given up, they would not have had any reason to celebrate him at last.

Have you noticed that those who try to discourage you are always the first to mock you the moment you finally give up? On the other hand, if you keep pushing regardless of the pressure from outside, a day will come when your naysayers will become announcers of your victory.

Lesson 8: He Threw Away His Coat.

Hearing that Jesus was calling him, Blind Bartimaeus immediately threw away his coat. As a beggar, the coat was probably his begging garment. Perhaps, the garment made it easier for people to identify him as a beggar. It could also be where he put the alms people gave him.

The Bible was not specific as to what he used the coat for. But whatever the coat meant to him, the good thing was that he knew quickly that he didn't want anything that would delay him from answering Jesus' call. He did not want anything that would stand as a barrier; hence, he needed to throw it away.

To you reading this, what is that thing that has become a burden and an extra load to you? It is time to lay them down at the feet of Jesus.

For some, it might be a sin you have allowed to come between you and your Maker. Today, would you come to Jesus, who can help you? Jesus has been calling you for ages, but that sin has held you back. It is time to let go.

Life is already too burdensome; why add extra load to yourself? Sin is an extra and unnecessary load. Unforgiveness, worry, grudges, greed, hatred, and bitterness are all extra and unnecessary loads. Why carry them when there is a Saviour to help you?

Be like Blind Bartimaeus, who threw away his extra load, jumped up, and went to meet Jesus.

Lesson 9: Jesus Asked Him A Question.

As I got to this part of the story, I felt uneasy. Why would Jesus be asking a poor blind man what he wanted? Could Jesus not see he was blind and needed his sight? At first, I felt the question was unnecessary, but as I brooded over it, I discovered that Jesus was right after all.

That he called out to Jesus for mercy does not necessarily mean he needed his sight back. People might assume that he needed his sight, not knowing that what he had in mind was for Jesus to give him alms. That is the essence of asking one what they specifically need.

Again, Jesus, being the Son of God, knew what the man wanted, but still allowed him to speak his mind because He wanted him to exercise his liberty to choose, and perhaps, He wanted a conversation with the man. This goes to show that Jesus does not discriminate. He can relate to anyone and everyone.

Jesus is not expecting you to pray about that situation confronting you because He is not aware of it, but He wants to interact with you. He desires a conversation with you. The delight you feel when your child asks you for anything is the same way God feels when His children trust Him enough to table their needs to Him.

Lesson 10: Blind Bartimaeus Knew What He Wanted

When Jesus asked what he wanted, he did not blab. He knew exactly what he wanted and went straight to the point.

He knew that if his sight was restored, other things could easily be sorted. With his eyes intact, he could stop begging and work with his hands.

What about you? If Jesus comes to you now to ask what you want, do you know that particular need that when sorted, other things will fall in place gradually?

Let me also point this out. The greatest need of every man is salvation. Do you already have that sorted? Think about it.

Lesson 11: He Received His Healing.

Jesus is so loving that He did not withhold healing from this man. That is how much

God loves humanity; it is how much God loves you. He loves you so much that He would never withhold anything good from you.

In the same way, Jesus gave this man what he wanted by healing him. He is also willing to help you today if you will let Him.

Lesson 12: He Followed Jesus.

The moment Jesus healed him, he did not say, *"Let me go home and mock those who have treated me badly in the past because of my blindness."* He did not try to prove a point to anyone. He followed Jesus immediately. He was so grateful that he could not let go of Jesus.

Many people today, when they are in trouble, will remember Jesus and run to Him for help, but immediately after their needs are met, they forget Him.

They only use God as a means to solve all their problems. They only remember God when they find themselves in trouble. But look at this man; he was so grateful that he had to follow Jesus immediately.

He did not use Jesus and dump Him as many people do today; he followed Him.

He recognised that what Jesus had done for him was what no other person could do for him and that Jesus was worth his following.

Dear reader, permit me to ask you, **"Are you among those who use and dump God?" "Have you truly decided to follow Jesus?"** I can tell you that Jesus is worth following.

Whether you acknowledge it or not, the truth is, God has been kind to you. It does not matter what you are currently going through, God has been good to you. He has done much for you that should make you pause and ponder His goodness.

Today, I encourage you to come to Jesus and follow Him. He is worth following. EMBRACE JESUS today. Bartimaeus did not only embrace the opportunity to be healed, but he also EMBRACED JESUS, his healer. Today, I encourage you to embrace Jesus. Tomorrow might be too late.

Chapter 6
Old Age – A Crown Or A Thorn?

"Ageing is not 'lost youth' but a new stage of opportunity and strength"
- Betty Friedan.

The fear of old age is a real fear. Many people are afraid of aging. For some, the thought of getting old someday scares them more than anything else.

But, whether you like it or not, and no matter how much you try to shy away from the subject of old age or the fact that you will get old someday, a time will come when you will no longer be able to run away from it because you are now face-to-face with the reality.

Old age is not a curse.

Old age is a blessing from God. But until you begin to view it from the lens of blessings, you will never stop feeling anxious or fretting at the thought or mention of it.

"I will satisfy him with long life and show him my salvation" is God's word of promise to His children in the book of Psalms 91:16. In other words, God is saying, *"I, the Lord will feed you with long life, you will eat it until you are old and satisfied and beyond that, I will show you my salvation and make you experience my saving power all through your life."* While living a long life, God will not leave you to figure out everything or fight everyday battles alone. Rather, as you go through life, He will be with you, deliver and save you from the power of sin, danger, and everything that stands as a threat to your life.

>
> "Do not regret growing older.
> It is a privilege denied to many."
> - Mark twain

It baffles me how people would spend time in religious houses praying for a long life and against anything that may try to cut their lives short, yet feel agitated when the topic of old age is raised. Isn't that an irony? Mark Twain wisely said, "Do not regret growing older. It is a privilege denied to many."

It also amazes me how many folks spend a lot to eat healthily, spend long hours exercising to stay fit, or spend almost all their earnings to celebrate birthdays but will almost pick a fight with anyone who reminds them of their age or that they are getting older. I thought the exercises, healthy eating, and prayers were to enable you to live long and healthy.

One of my friends once told me a true-life story of an older woman in her former area of residence. The woman would curse and pick a fight with anyone who greeted her and addressed her as 'Mama' or 'Mummy.' For instance, if a younger person greeted her in this manner, "Mama/Mummy, good morning," she would immediately pick a fight with the person, reminding the person that she was neither Mama nor Mummy but would gladly reply to anyone who called her 'Auntie.'

To that woman, calling her 'Mama' was a reminder that she was getting older and that was why she abhorred being called that. Contrarily, being referred to as 'Auntie' gave her the temporary feeling that she was young, even though in reality she was an older woman, probably, in her 70s.

As I grew older, I also suddenly began to feel odd about getting old. I had fearful thoughts ringing through my mind. I immediately knew that was fear of old age knocking. Knowing that if I didn't do anything about the fear, it would overwhelm me and probably get in the way of my happiness, I began to consciously reprogramme my mind by constantly reminding myself that it is a privilege to be alive. It is a privilege, not everyone has the opportunity to experience. By consciously reminding myself that, my mind gradually shifted from worrying to gratitude. That happened because I had started training my mind to see old age as a blessing from God.

Unfortunately, this fear of old age is not limited to people in their midlife or people of older generation. This fear also resides among people in their late twenties, thirties, and early forties. I noticed a certain fear that most people harbour while approaching thirty.

In life, fear is inevitable. As humans, we are prone to give in to fear occasionally. It is human to harbour fear about something, especially if it seems beyond our control. However, fear, when allowed to linger for too long, can become controlling and overly damaging.

The fear of old age, if not properly managed, can prevent you from living your best life. Uncontrolled fear is crippling.

If you don't learn how not to let fear of old age control you, you will have many things to regret when you finally reach there. While the fear of old age is real, overcoming it is also possible.

There are many reasons people harbour the fear of old age, but among many of them, there are two major reasons, which are peculiar to everyone, and those two reasons are what I want us to consider in the next few minutes.

Reasons For Fear Of Old Age

Underachievement: Underachievement is one of the reasons people tend to get agitated, anxious, or triggered whenever they remember that they are getting older.

Having examined and counselled many young people in their early thirties, I have realised why young people dread and become overly worried when approaching thirty because they feel their age does not match their achievements.

The same thing happens to every other age group. People become worried when they weigh their achievements against their age to see that things do not tally.

Diminished Youthfulness: The other day, I was returning from an event when I saw an older man in his 70s, a middle-aged woman, and a younger one standing side-by-side with him. One held him by his right hand and the other by his left.

The man looked feeble and sick, as he could barely walk. The women had to hold his hands to aid his walking. Even with the help from both women, the man still could not walk properly. His movement was so slow that one could see the struggle and pain he felt each time he lifted his legs.

As I walked past them, I turned around to look at them again, and this time, watching how the man struggled to walk. I felt pity for him.

Immediately, different thoughts ran through my mind. I said, "This is the old age we will all get to someday." Old age happens differently for everyone because while some become sick and feeble, others might be lucky to experience it without sickness or any of the many problems that follow aging.

But whichever way it happens, the truth is that just like that man in the above story, a time will come when you cannot walk as fast as you used to. A time will come when your eyes will no longer see as clearly as they used to, even though you are not blind. A time will come when meat will be staring at you in the face, and all you can do is look away because your teeth can no longer chew as they used to. A time will come when you will no longer be able to do the things you love to do today. After all, the vigour is no longer there, and this will be all thanks to old age.

The thought of watching our youthfulness evaporate is another reason people dread old age. Many people have not come to terms with the fact that they will not always be as strong or fresh as they are now. They do not want to imagine it because the thoughts are like having a nightmare.

How to Overcome the Fear of Old Age

Change Your Perspective: Perspective is how you see things in the eyes of your mind. It is the mindset you have formed about something based on what you consistently expose your mind to. Concisely, perspective is how your mind views and interprets a thing, which determines how you react or respond to it.

People are not scared of old age because they have been old before and have experienced what and how it feels to be old. Most people who dread old age are not old yet. They are usually young folks who have allowed their minds to view old age from the lens of negativity.

For many others, their fear stems from their experience living and caring for their old parents, grandparents, or relatives. Having witnessed firsthand how old age dealt with those people, their perspective of old age became completely altered.

I once had the privilege of caring for my aged grandmother, and I can admit that the experience was challenging. There were frequent instances when I needed to clean her and her room due to incontinence. Every night, while others prayed for sustenance and protection, she would pray to God to take her life, feeling weary of her situation and longing for relief from her physical confinement.

If I had not consciously worked on my mindset, my experience of caring for my grandmother could have distorted my perspective on old age and instilled fear in me. That is why it is essential to consistently renew your mind and intentionally train it to see ageing as a blessing rather than a curse.

Indeed, it is a huge blessing to go through childhood, teenagehood, and adulthood and still have the golden privilege to reach old age. Everyone wishes for this privilege regardless of fear. Yet, it is not everyone who gets the opportunity to experience it.

Old age, though burdensome and limiting in some ways, is never a curse or a thorn. It is a blessing. Only God can put on you this crown of old age. I used to dread it, too. But one of the things that have helped me overcome the fear is that I began to make a conscious effort to train my mind to view and respond to the thought of it as a crown rather than a thorn.

Old age is a beautiful crown that only God can bestow upon you. Therefore, embrace it and cherish it. When you reach that stage in life, treasure it and enjoy it to the fullest.

Be Like Jesus: *"I must work the works of Him who sent me while it is day; the night* *is coming when no one can work." John 9:4 (NKJV).*

Instead of sitting and brooding over old age and all the troubles that accompany it, why not be like Jesus? Jesus was a man who understood His assignment on earth. Beyond understanding His assignment, He also understood something called 'night.' His understanding of this fact helped him embrace every moment and kept Him on His toes to be about the work He came to earth to do.

Even though Jesus knew that night would come, which in His case was Death on the Cross, He did not focus on the night. He did not burden or worry Himself with that. Rather, He chose to focus on doing the work God had assigned Him to do and to ensure its completion before night came.

Night for you and me could mean old age, illness, death, or the Second Coming of Christ. When any of the above happens, doing any work will be impossible or near impossible. Hence, instead of focusing on the fact that night (old age) would come, when you will no longer be able to go about your assignment or to do the things you love, why not be like Jesus and focus on doing those things now so that when your night finally comes you can beat your chest in excitement and fulfilment and say like Apostle Paul,

"I have fought a good fight, I have finished my course, I have kept the faith?" 2 Timothy 4:7 (KJV).

There is no greater pain than getting old and having many things to regret. Regret makes old age more daunting and burdensome.

If you commit yourself today to embracing each moment and doing what truly matters, you will have little or no time to worry about old age. Give yourself fully to serving your generation. Make the most of your life every day, and see how your fears will dissipate.

How to Evade Regret in Old Age

Prepare for It: Many people do not plan or prepare for old age. That is why when it knocks at their door, they dread it because they have many things they wished they had done better.

Most people plan for their marriage, childbearing, and so on, but very few plan for their old age. The truth is, you will not always be young and strong. You will not always be able to lift heavy items and run around as you used to. What are you doing today to prepare for the days when your vigour is no longer there?

"The future belongs to those who prepare for it today" - Malcolm X. The future does not belong to everyone. It only belongs to those who spend their today prepping for it.

Old age is not something you suddenly wake up to. It is something you walk into gradually. Hence, if you spend your day worrying about old age instead of preparing for it, you will arrive there, only to find out that you have no enjoyable place in it.

There is a saying, "You cannot feature in a future you do not picture." Old age is something that you must first picture in the eyes of your mind and how you want it to be before beginning to plan and prepare for it by maximising all that God has put in you.

Picture yourself in your 60s, 70s, 80s, 90s, and even 100-plus years, depending on how long you wish to be here and how you wish your life to be. Then, prayerfully prepare for it. Whether or not you will live up to that age should not bother you, as that is not in your power to do.

Just PICTURE, PLAN, and PRAY about your desire while maximising today.

Live Meaningfully: One of the things that will help you not to end up in regrets in old age is knowing that you lived for God and that you truly gave life your all.

At the end of your life, of course, you already know that in a normal situation, old age is the final phase before transitioning to the other side of eternity. When you get to that phase of your life where you are old and feeble, it will no longer matter much to you how many houses you built or the amount of wealth you have acquired.

It may not matter much to you how many countries you have travelled to, the certificates you have acquired, or even the number of children you have. These things, as important as they are, may not matter much to you. That is because you can have all that and more and still live with regrets.

The things that will make more sense to you or even give your old age meaning and leave you fulfilled will be the services you rendered to God and humanity.

Living purposefully is one sure way to make your old age worthwhile. You have not truly lived until your life becomes a medium through which others are helped or why others find reasons to live too.

Life in itself is meaningless. Only your love for God and service to Him through your services to humanity give life meaning. As such, loving God and serving His purposes in your younger years give value and meaning to your older years.

Old age is a privilege denied to many. You have to prepare for it and embrace it fully.

Chapter 7
Foes In Friends' Cloak

"True enemies are better than false friends."
– Matshona Dhliwayo.

In my over 30 years of serving in God's vineyard as a counsellor, minister of the Word, and one who has had to encourage people from different walks of life and backgrounds, I have had the golden privilege of people confiding in me about many issues eating them up. I can tell you that one of the major issues people have had to confide in me about is betrayal by family members, lovers, friends, colleagues, or just people they once trusted. That is to say, people close to you are usually the ones who betray you, not those far from you.

The issue of foes in friends' garments is a real issue many are battling with. Many people are not who they appear to be or whom people perceive them as.

Moreover, many folks today carry the burden of pains inflicted on them directly or indirectly by the people they loved and trusted. This pain can cut so deep that the victims, not knowing how best to handle the situation, can become not only devastated but depressed and, in some cases, suicidal.

Sometime ago, the news was making rounds on the internet about a young and beautiful lady who took her life after being jilted by her fiancé of many years. Unfortunately, this lady's case is just one out of many. Many people are hurting due to betrayal from people they love and trust.

Friendship should be taken seriously; many people are so careless in choosing their friends. Not everyone who crosses your path is worth being your friend.

You should have a standard for measuring and choosing your friends. There are people you should never bring too close to your life. You should only love them from afar.

There are people who, no matter how nicely they present themselves, you should never let into the 'holy of holies' of your life. They can remain at the 'outer court' until you have genuinely proven they are worth being in your 'inner chamber.'

Indeed, we can never be too careful as people change for good or bad. People you see as good today can, in later years, be worse than some you consider as bad.

However, applying caution will shield you from carrying many potential foes in your boat.

In this chapter, I will be taking you through three major topics – types of friends, how to discern real/unreal friends, and how to handle betrayal

Types of Friends

Here, I will explain the kinds of people you may encounter as friends and how to identify them:

Frenemies: These are the real foes in friends' cloak. They are enemies disguised as friends and have never considered you as friends before. They are not friends who change to foes over time.

Such people are enemies on a deadly mission who come into your life with evil intentions from the beginning but pretend to be friends. They have their evil mission planned out from the onset. However, for them to achieve their desire, they first pose as friends. But they are never one.

Frenemies can go the extra mile to get at you even if it means discomforting themselves for a while. If it means acting all nice around you just to get at you, they will do it. If it means going out of their way to help you, they will do it.

Frenemies can do anything to make you loosen up to them. This could mean relocating to your city, applying to work in your company, or begging you to accommodate them in your home for a while. To convince you to accommodate them, they can form being stranded. They can just do anything to make you pity them and draw them close enough to monitor you and strike during your vulnerable moments.

The easiest way to see beyond the physical acts of such people is to have a discerning spirit.

Breezy Friends: This set of friends only remembers you when they have a need that they feel you can meet. They can go on for weeks or even months without calling or texting you to say 'Hello.' They hardly check up on you but only remember your address or contact when they need help.

I call them breezy friends because they only breeze in when they need you and breeze out if you are not relevant. These friends may not necessarily have bad intentions towards you, but because they see you as a means to an end, they can become dangerously entitled and bitter whenever you try to say no to their demands.

Conditional Friends: These friends are known as good-time friends. As long as you have the money and are ready to spend it, you are healthy enough to hang out with them when they want, you are highly placed in society, you bring something to the table, honey flows from your end, and there is benefit of attaching themselves to your life, then they are good to go.

These friends are usually the first to desert you when the going gets tough because their friendship with you is conditional.

Destiny Friends: These are the kind of friends that the Bible refers to as friends that stick closer than a brother (Proverbs 18:24). They are friends who have become like family because of how they always look out for you.

These friends are not easy to come by. But when you find one, you can always count on them. They are real friends.

Destiny friends, rejoice when you rejoice and cry when you cry. They are the ones who stand by you and with you, lending their shoulders for you to cry on and helping to wipe your tears when the need arises. They have your best interest at heart and are always willing to share with you and correct you in love when you err.

These friends are not there to only wine and dine with you; they are strategically positioned in your life to support you as you fulfil your destiny.

How to Discern Real Friends

Here are top ways to identify friends who will be there for you:

Does Not Demean Your Win: One of the ways to know a real friend is how they celebrate your win, including your little wins. A real friend will always rejoice with you when you are rejoicing and does not demean you or talk down on your achievements, no matter how small they are.

Even if it is just something as little as overcoming a heartbreak, walking out of a toxic relationship, learning a new language, earning an extra paycheck, gaining or losing weight, whatever it is, as long as you consider it a win, a real friend should be able to celebrate with you and cheer you on to achieve more.

Any friend who frowns at you celebrating a little win is not a real friend but a dangerous one. If you are not trying to hide under the guise of celebration to mock them or others, then I don't see any reason they should not be happy for you.

A real friend is genuinely happy for you when you are winning. With this parameter, you can also judge yourself to know if you are a real friend to your friends, too.

Does Not Try To Snatch Your Moment: Have you ever accomplished a feat or has something good happened to you, and while you are trying to share your good news with your friend(s), they suddenly interrupt you? They steer the conversation away from you and go, *"Oh yeah, that reminds me, last week I won a new contract. My boss just gave me a raise. My fiancé just got me a new Gucci handbag, shoes, and a wristwatch."*

Now, that is an unreal friend. A genuine friend will listen to you share your good news, and celebrate with you wholeheartedly without trying to snatch the moment by interrupting you with their stories to prove that you are not the only one winning.

Why have they not shared their 'good news' with you all along? Why wait until you want to share yours to interrupt with theirs? Okay, assuming they forgot to tell you earlier, the right thing to do would have been to listen to you, as you share your wins and then, celebrate with you. Later, they can share their achievements with you so you can celebrate with them.

Does Not Stand With The Crowd Against You: Your real friends are the ones who will never stand with the crowd against you even if you are wrong. They do not even have to support your wrongdoing to prove their solidarity. Rather, they condemn your wrongdoing in love while protecting you from the mob.

Does Not Keep Records Of Offenses: It is in human nature to disagree. Misunderstandings are inevitable; even in marital relationships, couples still disagree on certain issues. Therefore, it is not out of place to respectfully disagree with your friends sometimes. Note the word 'respectfully' because even while disagreeing with others, you can still maintain some level of decorum and respect for their person. However, when you have a friend who always keeps records of offenses to the point where they start bearing grudges and becoming malicious over every misunderstanding, and goes as far as turning those records into a weapon in the future, that is already a red flag.

Real friends do not keep records of offenses. Rather, they find ways to iron things out and settle them amicably while doing all they can to avoid a recurrence.

Does Not Pressure You Unnecessarily: There are times in life when pressure becomes necessary. For instance, a friend can take it upon themself not to allow you to feel comfortable in mediocrity. With that in mind, they can go the extra mile to challenge you to level up through skill upgrading or personal development, while also allowing you some reasonable amount of space to grow at your pace without overwhelming you.

Notwithstanding, if you have a friend who constantly pressures you unnecessarily, especially when the velocity at which they are moving is discomforting and leading you into anxiety and dangerous behaviours, then it is time to stay away from such a person.

For instance, if a friend thinks you are too cheap because you are not wearing designer clothes and pressures you to level up by buying expensive wear without considering if you can afford it, that's a very dangerous friend to watch out for.

As long as what you wear is what you can afford, and as long as you always dress decently and neatly, I see no reason a friend should not be okay with it. This kind of unhealthy pressure is the reason many young women are going into prostitution and young men are becoming dubious simply because they want to "feel among." A real friend who values you will not pressure you into wrongdoing.

Does Not Make You Feel Less: Have you ever had a friend or currently have a close friend who constantly brings you down, either directly or indirectly? If your answer to the above question is a yes, I put it to you that the person is a threat to your destiny.

A real friend uplifts you not just with their words but through their actions as well. They point you to your good qualities and abilities, celebrate you, and cheer you on. They also help you see the good in you, your hidden talents, and everything that makes you amazing by always amplifying them. A real friend does not hesitate to encourage you to work on the areas you are not measuring up yet.

On the contrary, an unreal friend will always try to belittle your good qualities and talents. They never see anything good in you. They do everything within their power to water down your potential but will always amplify your weakness. That's because their goal is to deflate your self-worth, because by so doing, you will continue to feel less of yourself.

The dangerous thing about keeping such people around you is that it will get to a point where you will begin to define yourself by their negative opinions of you. Unfortunately, this can lead you into self-hatred manifesting in all kinds of deviant behaviours. Your real friend can never make you feel less of yourself.

Does Not Drain Your Energy Through Negativity: Next to friends who make you feel less are those who constantly sap your energy through negativity.

These kinds of people are full of negative energy. They are carriers of bad news and impossibilities. They are the ones who always see why an idea will not work out. They are those friends who will point you to reasons they think something might go wrong. For this set of friends, even when they cannot see any impossibility, they will create one. Their major objective is to discourage you and drain your enthusiasm so you do not get to try.

Real friends are the ones, who even if they can see challenges ahead, will help you figure out ways to navigate it because they want to see you dare your fears and go for your goals.

Does Not Disrespect Boundaries: Some friends can be nosy and want to know everything happening in your life. It is important to be aware of friends who constantly pry into your personal matters despite your efforts to keep certain details private. While they may appear to be caring, their motives could be questionable. Be cautious around such individuals, as they may pose a potential risk to you and your loved ones.

Real friends recognise and respect boundaries. Imagine a friend, visiting your home and going straight to your kitchen to dish out food, even when you have made it clear that you do not like people crossing such boundaries. A true friend should always ask for permission before doing certain things in your house. Some people may not mind others going through their things as they please, but if it is a deal-breaker for you, others should respect it. Another scenario is this: if you experience a situation you would prefer not to talk about, your friends should respect that decision.

Does Not Compete With You: Have you ever met competitive friends? They are one of the worst kinds of friends to have.

Such friends always want to prove they are better than you. They may not say it but the subtle behaviour of constant comparison proves that the person competes with you.

Real friends collaborate. Real friends complement each other, not compete.

When you have friends who always compare their achievements with yours or themselves with you, it is time to free yourself from such bondage. A competitive fellow can go the extra mile to prove they are better, even if it means hurting you.

Does Not Trash-Talk You Before Others: This one is the hallmark of a dangerous friend. A person who goes behind you to talk bad about you or even fabricate lies against you just to get others to hate you is the definition of an unreal friend.

If you have that kind of person in your life, it is high time you dissociate from them because being in that unhealthy environment can be detrimental to you.

Real friends do not trash-talk each other.

How to Handle Betrayal from Friends

If a friend betrays you, the next step is to seek ways to heal. Here, I will outline ways to make that happen:

Do Not Live in Denial of the Betrayal: Refusing to acknowledge or accept that you have been betrayed by someone you trust is one sure way to never heal from the hurt.

Living in denial is usually the first way people respond to grief. However, if you continue to live in denial, you will only end up hurting yourself more.

The betrayal might have come from someone you never thought would ever hurt you. The fact that you thought that person could never hurt you is the more reason you are in pain and cannot come to terms with the reality that the person has betrayed you.

But if you truly desire to heal from the pain and move on with your life, accepting what had happened is your sure bet to healing. Not accepting the reality early enough will only prolong your pain unnecessarily.

Let Out Your Emotions: Bottling up hurts creates room for more hurts. The more you try to bottle up your emotions, the more you inflict pain on yourself.

Let it out. If you have to cry, do so. If you have to vent, it is cool. But ensure that in letting out your emotion, you do not go overboard by using weapon or deadly substances on yourself. Suicide has never solved problems for anyone and will not solve yours.

This is why I encourage people to confide in someone when betrayal happens. Vent to a trusted person whom you feel comfortable with and who will not judge you.

Do not Be Too Hard On Yourself: Usually, when betrayal happens, you might become angry with yourself. Perhaps you opened a door of your life for the wrong person, or you let out information about yourself to the person you thought would never do you wrong, only to find out later that you were wrong. The thought of that can lead you to self-blame, but you must understand it was not your fault. Even if it was, you need to forgive yourself.

Being too hard on yourself will make it harder to heal from that betrayal. Remember that the deed has been done and you cannot turn back the hand of the clock.

Engage in Physical Exercises: One of the ways I handle pain is to take a long walk. Even when I'm angry about something, taking a long walk can calm my nerves and help me see things the way they are. It also gives me direction on how to respond to the issue without hurting myself more or letting things get out of hand.

Some people prefer to take a long sleep. Sleep, as a form of exercise, is therapeutic and helps to cool your head. When you wake up, you can look into the situation again. This time, you will look at it from a positive perspective.

Exercise can get you in the right mood and help you overcome a difficult situation.

Do not Give Room to Retaliation: When a friend betrays you, the worst way to handle the betrayal is to give in to revenge.

Revenge has never solved anyone's problem; instead, it worsens it. Though at first, retaliation may make you feel good because you think that by making the person feel the pains you are feeling, you will feel better. Sadly, that is not true. Retaliation leaves you worse off in the end.

You cannot solve an existing problem by creating more problems. Retaliation is equivalent to creating more problems for yourself. Inflicting pain on those who have betrayed you will never take away the pain of the betrayal. Hence, revenge will not help you find the peace and healing you truly need.

After a betrayal, you need healing. Resorting to revenge will hamper the process.

Distance Yourself: Remaining close to the person who has betrayed you is unhealthy for you.

You must stay far from them and avoid any conversation where they will be the subject matter. This will foster your healing process. Besides, it is different from keeping malice with them. If you can't completely avoid the person, you can maintain a healthy boundary or simply reduce your interaction to only greetings. Anything beyond that, mind your business.

Forgive: This is one of the most challenging things to do, especially if the offender does not care that they have done you wrong.

Without forgiveness, you will not be able to heal. Forgiveness facilitates your healing.

Forgiveness precedes healing.

Forgiveness fosters healing.

That you forgave a person does not mean what they did to you was right. It means you love yourself and value yourself enough not to let their acts of irresponsibility hinder you from moving on. It means that you prioritise your well-being over their wickedness. It means you understand that your life, health, and general well-being matter more to you.

Forgiveness also improves your health. According to experts, it can lower heart rates/blood pressure, and reduce anxiety, which can lead to depression and improve your heart health.

Forgiveness is the easiest way to heal from betrayal.

Learn from What Happened: This is very important. No matter how bad an experience is, there is always a lesson you can glean from it if you pay attention.

Learning from whatever life throws at you is necessary. With the lessons you glean from what happened, you can refrain from allowing a recurrence. Then, you can chart a new path for your life and destiny.

In summary, learn how to discern. With discernment, you can tell when a friend is tilting towards becoming dangerous to you.

This is why it is necessary to have a personal relationship with the Holy Spirit. There are things that no matter how much you try, you will never decipher by your human wisdom, except God makes you privy to it by revelation or discernment.

The Holy Spirit can also help us make the right choice of friends if we let Him. He desires to help us but can only do so if we let Him.

Imagine how many wrong people you might have to carry in your boat of destiny if God does not help you discern who is worth journeying with you. Imagine how many people might betray you if you keep depending on your human wisdom for something the Holy Spirit can help you prevent.

Carrying the wrong people in your boat can prevent you from fully embracing every moment of your life. I pray you heal from whatever betrayal you have faced.

EMBRACE EVERY MOMENT

Chapter 8
I Am Single, So What?

"Singleness is no longer a lack of option - but a choice - a choice to refuse to let your life be defined by your relationship status but to live every day Happily and let your Ever After work itself out"
- Mandy Hale.

While writing this book, I felt a leading to write to my single sons and daughters and every single person who will come across this book. At first, I tried to wave it aside with the excuse that it is not a relationship book. Nevertheless, as I delved deeper into birthing the book, the nudge grew stronger that I could no longer overlook it.

In my many years of working as a counsellor, I have had the opportunity to counsel many single men and women. From my interaction with them, I can tell that people's perspective and approach to singlehood differ from individual to individual.

While some bask in the euphoria of singleness, enjoying, building, and making the most of their singlehood, others just brood along as though being single is an affliction.

Being single is not easy. It comes with many untold challenges. However, the challenge does not negate that singleness is a blessing.

I have heard and seen folks mock people for being single as though singleness is a crime. People tend to stigmatise the singles as if there is something particularly wrong with them for not being married. Sometimes, I can't help but wonder how people shame their fellow humans for a phase that everyone must go through.

Singlehood is a phase, just like every other phase in life. No one is ever born married. Even the married person today was once single. So, why try to talk down on people and make them feel bad for something, not within their control?

"There is an appointed time for everything and a time for every affair under the heavens" - *Ecclesiastes 3:1 (New American Bible).*

As the scripture above states, there is a time and a season for every affair and activity under the sun. Singleness is only a phase; a season that will come and go when the appointed time comes.

What I find distressing is that many people have been pressured too much about marriage and made to think that their lives had little or no meaning outside of it. Painfully, many unmarried people have allowed such to lead them into pausing their lives with the mindset that their lives will start making meaning when they are finally married. The effect of it is that it has made some single folks not truly live; they merely exist.

Dear singles, let me remind you that your life does not start when you are married. Your life has started, and you have to start living. Chase your dreams, discover yourself, enrol for a training, go back to school, learn a skill, start a business, and ensure that you are truly living and not just sitting with folded arms waiting for marriage to find you.

Get busy and let marriage meet you being productive at your duty post. Waiting to be married before chasing your dreams is wasting your singlehood. Singleness is like currency; invest it wisely. Whatever you invest in your singlehood, you will reap in marriage. Marriage is a harvesting ground for the seeds you sowed while single. Are you sowing wisely or foolishly? Ponder that.

Will Everyone Get Married?

Most people always avoid this part of the conversation about singleness.

The thought that not everyone will get married scares many to death. No matter how scary it sounds or how uncomfortable it makes you feel, the truth remains that not everyone will get married.

For some, the decision not to get married is their personal choice. But others, for reasons beyond their control, will find out that marriage doesn't seem to happen for them. This is a fact that everyone has to make peace with.

Making peace with this assertion does not connote that if you encounter disappointments in a relationship or are not married at a certain age, you are not destined to be married. Rather, it means that while you desire marriage, you should also not allow the thought about whether you will ever get married or not to weigh you down. It means that you should give yourself the fulfilment of your purpose to the point where you don't have time to worry about whether you are destined for marriage or not. This, too, is a great way to live above desperation.

Wisdom for Single Men/Women

We live in a couple-oriented society where one of the most applauded statuses is to have the tag "wife/husband" to your name.

I Am Single, So What?

For most people, singleness comes with a series of emotional rollercoasters. This moment, they are high on positivity; the next moment, they swim in the abyss of worthlessness because they think their lives are meaningless outside marriage.

Marriage is beautiful, and I pray that everyone who desires it will get an opportunity to experience it. However, marriage will not automatically add meaning to your life if you have always considered your life meaningless as a single fellow.

You can live a meaningful life as a single as much as you can also live a meaningful life as a married person. In other words, singleness is not synonymous with meaninglessness. Likewise, being married is not synonymous with meaningfulness.

Dear single, your marital status does not increase or reduce your worth, nor does it define who you are. What you do with your life every day does. Hence, the big question is, "What are you doing with your life now?"

Now that you are single, are you investing in your personal development or are you busy complaining and wailing about not being married? No matter how you look at it, singlehood has several advantages, but many don't see them.

Freedom

One of the biggest advantages of singleness is the freedom that comes with it. Note that freedom here is not about having the liberty to do whatever you want without considering its consequences. It is not about going wherever you want and coming back anytime you deem fit without being accountable to anyone. Rather, it is the liberty to invest your time wisely in developing yourself and honing your skills.

Now that you are single is the best time to learn a skill, acquire a certification, apply for training, etc. There are so many things that freedom of singlehood can afford you.

The reason you have enough time to worry about your marital status is that you have not given yourself any valuable course. You think marriage is all there is to your life. That is not true. There is more that God wants to do with your life. Marriage could be one of them, but not all.

As a single man/woman to be married someday, have you discovered God's purpose for your life? Have you understood the problem God put you on earth to solve? Even if marriage is all that God created you to do, do you know that now that you are single is the right time to build and prepare yourself for that assignment?

Even marriage needs preparation. You cannot wake up any day and jump into it. Therefore, now is the best time to start preparing for it. Many things are there to invest your time as a single man/woman rather than just wasting away in worry and wailing.

How to Make the Most of Your Singleness

To enjoy a fulfilling singleness, you need to incorporate the following into your waiting period:

Accountability

Now that you are single is a great time to learn accountability. I know you can do whatever you want without anyone questioning you. Contrarily, it would be foolish to think that being single negates accountability.

It is important to have a trusted person you can be accountable to. This will help put you in check in case you want to derail.

Live Joyfully

Living without physical intimacy or a romantic relationship yet being happy through the process is a skill every single man/woman must learn.

I know you feel lonely sometimes. I understand there are days when your heart yearns to have a heart-to-heart conversation with a man/woman of your own. Still, in the absence of all that, you can train yourself to find reasons to be happy.

Do the Things You Love

Doing the things you love is a great way to make your singlehood interesting. It can bring a level of fulfilment. Engaging in activities that interest you is a helpful way to distract yourself from the worrying thoughts of singlehood. Any time you spend doing the things you love is never wasted.

Invest in Your Personal Development

The importance of investing in you can never be overemphasized. Life is designed in such a way that you can only attract certain things as you grow. Growth can never happen outside of investment in you.

Many only sit back, waiting and hoping for marriage to happen. They never make time to invest in themselves, forgetting that only the developed version of themselves can handle the challenges that accompany marriage when it finally happens.

It is an aberration and an injustice against yourself if you deny yourself an opportunity to grow due to your inability to invest correctly in yourself today. As a single, do you create time to read transformational books? Do you create time to attend seminars and conferences? Do you take professional certification and training for your career? Have you thought of upgrading your financial life? What do you use your time for?

Pondering these questions is crucial to your growth. Read quality books, attend conferences, build destiny relationships, invest in your looks, learn a new skill, apply for training to up your game in business/career, and go back to school if you have to. Ensure you don't abandon yourself. Do something every day that improves your life.

Embrace Every Moment

One mistake I have observed in many singles is that they tend to put their lives on hold until they get married. It is important to understand that your life has already started the moment you were born, and waiting for marriage to happen is not the way to live it. Thus, it would be unwise to hit the pause button on your life, hoping to replay it once you tie the knot.

EMBRACE EVERY MOMENT

Live your life fully and live it now. Embrace every moment you have to live with gratitude, enthusiasm, and hard work. Living in the moment means you do not postpone anything until you are married. Do the things you have to do today. Leave no stone unturned in ensuring that your life counts today.

Chapter 9
The Deceit Of Youthfulness

"A good youth ought to have a fear of God, to be subject to his parents, to give honour to his elders, to preserve his purity; he ought not to despise humility, but should love forbearance and modesty. All these are an ornament to youthful years."
- **Saint Ambrose.**

The youthful phase is interesting. It is an important stage in a person's life. It is so important that its importance can never be overemphasized. Being young is an advantage. To be young is like having a great asset at your disposal.

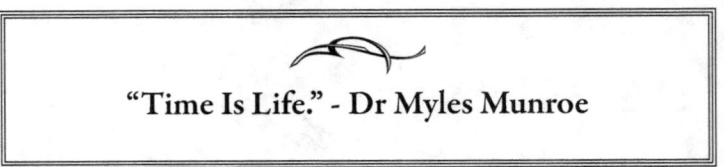

"Time Is Life." - Dr Myles Munroe

But unfortunately, many youths today do not understand the importance of youthfulness and the fact that it is a fleeting stage. Like every other thing that is subject to change, it does not last. Many young people today erroneously believe that they have all the time in the world to mess around and still return to doing the things that truly matter to their lives and destinies.

I have seen many videos on social media about young people bragging about how they have the right to live their lives whichever way they want and do whatever they want because, to them, *"we are young and can afford to do whatever we want."*

They do not yet realise that they can never recover every minute they squander on doing irrelevant things. In the words of Dr. Myles Munroe, *"Time Is Life."* In other words, anytime you spend your time doing unimportant things, you are indirectly and unknowingly wasting your life.

Many young people today squander their youthfulness on things that add no value to them or others. Funnily enough, they often think they can return to make things right. They forget that any time they lost has indeed been lost. They also do not know that not every age is convenient for doing certain things. Some things are age-applicable. The youthful years are a time to build your life. Does this mean people can no longer build their lives in old age? That is not what I am saying. However, can you imagine a 70-year-old man returning to primary school or learning a new skill for business purposes? Can you compare that older man's efficiency and concentration to that of a younger person? While there are instances of people achieving remarkable feats in their older age, it's a drop in the ocean compared to the number who got it right in their youth.

The Bible also established that *"It is good for a man that he bears the yoke in his youth." - Lamentation 3:27.* This goes to expand what Apostle Joshua Selman said in his message titled, *'Maximising Destiny'* that *"Every time is not convenient for everything."*

Truly, not every time is convenient for everything, which is why the Bible encourages people to bear their yoke in their youth. This means that the youthful stage is not a time to do just anything that presents itself. It is a time to invest your time consciously and wisely into building your life. There are things you should not invest your youthfulness in, and there are things you should invest your youthfulness in.

One thing I aim to achieve in this chapter is to bring you to a point where you begin to value your youthfulness and understand that the stage is also a currency with which you buy a great future for yourself. Armed with that notion, you can begin to invest your youthfulness wisely. Do not waste it. It is a precious time many are regretting not taking proper advantage of. What about you, basking in the euphoria of youthfulness? Are you maximising it?

There are things you should never spend your youthfulness on, and there are things you should not hesitate to spend it on. Before I share with you a few ways to invest your youthfulness wisely to attain a great life, let me remind you of some things you should never invest your youthfulness in.

EMBRACE EVERY MOMENT

Your youthfulness should not be invested in experimenting with sexual immoralities.

Your youthfulness should not be invested in building bad behaviours.

Your youthfulness should not be invested in crime of any kind.

Your youthfulness should not be invested in laziness, procrastination, and complacency.

Your youthfulness should not be invested in the wrong association.

Your youthfulness should not be invested in rumour-mongering.

Your youthfulness should not be invested in creating enemies for yourself due to your bad and unholy lifestyle.

Your youthfulness should not be invested in displeasing God.

Think about anything that does not align with the will of God for your life, or that does not propel you into serving the purposes of God and living life to the fullest. Those are the things you should never invest your youthfulness into.

If you invest in the above-listed, you cannot expect the same result as someone who invested appropriately. Your investment determines your returns.

Now, what are the things you should invest in? Let me bring in the quote at the opening of this chapter, and with that, I will show you how to invest your youthfulness wisely.

"A good youth ought to have the fear of God, to be subject to his parents, to give honour to his elders, to preserve his purity; he ought not to despise humility, but should

love forbearance and modesty. All these are an ornament to youthful years."

Ought to Have the Fear of God:

"The fear of the Lord, the Bible says, is the beginning of wisdom, and knowledge of the Holy One, an understanding. For through me, your days will be many and years will be added to your life." Proverbs 9:10-11 (NIV).

A youth who reverences and fears God is wise. Many youths today despise God and the things of God. From the scripture above, a youth who despises God is synonymous with foolishness. It is in having reverence for God that you become wise, and it is equally in doing so that your days will be multiplied and years added to your life. With this, you can see that you lose nothing by being a godly youth who fears God.

Ought to be Subject to His/Her Parents: You cannot despise your parents and expect to attain a life of honour. It is in honouring your parents that you will be honoured. I have come across young people who despise, disrespect, and treat their parents with disdain. They do not know that by doing so, they bring curses on themselves and incur the wrath of God. There is a saying that your parents are your earthly god. If you honour God and dishonour your parents, God will not be pleased with you. He demands that while you honour Him, you should do the same to your parents. You did not choose your parents; God did. It is not by mistake that you have them as your parents, and God requires you to cherish them and submit to them in obedience.

Ought to Give Honour to His/Her Elders: Honour for your elders is very important. If you fear God and honour your parents but despise your elders, you are still an unwise youth. The youth who despises his elders is already wishing not to become one. Youthfulness invested in fearing God, submitting to parents, and honouring the elders is never a waste.

Ought to Preserve His/Her Purity: The youth who upholds purity is a youth who will achieve much in life. Impurity is a destroyer of life and destiny. If, as a youth, you detest purity, you will see yourself engaging in much regrettable behaviour. Purity, in every form, is required of any youth who truly desires to attain a meaningful life. Purity entails that you uphold honesty, live a transparent life, eschew evil, be of godly conduct and character, think purely, abstain from sexual immoralities, et cetera. You can never go wrong by living a pure life.

Ought Not to Despise Humility: Humility is required of any youth who desires a life of honour and greatness. *"But He gives more grace. Therefore, He says: God resists the proud, but gives grace to the humble." James*

4:6 (NKJV). When God resists you, nothing else works in your life. This is why it is vital to live a humble life to avoid incurring the resistance of God. Humility is necessary for your rising.

To fear God, submit to your earthly parents, and honour your elders, all required some level of purity. Beyond that, if you truly want to grow in any facet of your life, you must be humble. Be humble enough to learn, submit to authorities, admit being wrong when you make mistakes, ask questions when you don't understand something, and do the right things. The importance of humility to your rising can never be overemphasized.

Ought to Love Forbearance: Forbearance is your ability to exercise self-control, restraint, and tolerance under great provocation. Any youth who lacks self-control is defenceless. Self-control is a shield to anyone who has it. *"A person without* *self-control is like a city with broken-down walls." Proverbs 25:28 (NLT).*

This scripture above explains how defenceless a lack of self-control can make one. As a young person, you will come across situations where you will be greatly provoked and your patience tested. At such times, one of the things that can keep you from making deadly mistakes or doing things that you might live the rest of your life regretting will be your ability to apply self-restraint.

Ought to Love Modesty: A youth who learns to do things in moderation has learned a good way of life. Going overboard on anything can be dangerous. Learn to be moderate in everything, and see yourself living more meaningfully.

These ornaments make youthfulness beautiful. There is no beauty in waywardness and rascality. Only by doing these things can your youthfulness be fully maximised.

"Remember now you were Creator in the days of your youth before the difficult days come, and the years draw near, when you say, "I have no pleasure in them" Ecclesiastics 12:1 (NKJV).

Up there are the most reasonable ways to invest your youthfulness. To think you can live your youthful years messing around and still have enough time to come back and correct your actions is just one of the deceits of youthfulness.

Remember your creator now that you are young. Invest your youthfulness into serving Him and making the most of your life. You cannot invest your youthfulness in wrongdoings and expect the same result as another who invested theirs in pleasing God and developing themselves.

EMBRACE EVERY MOMENT

You will not always be young. Therefore, wisdom demands that you spend your youthfulness on things that will impact you meaningfully.

The youthful years are your sowing years. Hence, whatever you do now is a seed you are sowing, which you must harvest someday. The big question is, are you sowing wisely or foolishly? Youthfulness lost can never be regained. This is the reason you should apply your heart to wisdom.

Dear youth,
As you embrace every moment of your life, do not forget to embrace your youthfulness and make the most of it.

Chapter 10

The Ungrateful Thorn: Rising Above The Pain Of Ingratitude

"Even though many people prove to be ungrateful, do not let that stop you from benefiting others - for not only is beneficence in itself a noble and almost divine quality, it may also happen that while you practice it, you will encounter someone so grateful that he will make up for all the others' ingratitude"
- **Francesco Guicciardini.**

In a world where kindness is often seen as a currency, the story of betrayal and ingratitude strikes a resonant chord. This chapter delves into the heart-wrenching experiences of those who have extended their hands in aiding and servicing of others, only to have them bitten by the souls they sought to uplift.

What you are about to read is a narrative of resilience, a testament to the strength of the human spirit in the face of duplicity and ungratefulness. As we navigate these stories, we are reminded of the biblical verse from Luke 6:35, *"But love your enemies, do good to them, and lend to them without expecting to get anything back."* This profound scripture encourages us to persist in our kindness, regardless of the outcome, emphasizing the virtue of unconditional generosity.

Humanly speaking, this is hard to do. Imagine offering help to a fellow who once talked badly about you to others, spreading falsehood against you, not minding how helpful you have always been to them. Imagine praying for a family member who once mocked you. Imagine being there for a friend who was nowhere to be found when you needed them the most. It is hard to do. However, we draw strength from the Apostle Paul's proclamation, *"I can do all things through Christ who strengthens me."*

"You may encounter many defeats,
but you must not be defeated."
- Maya Angelou.

Many of us have felt the sting of ingratitude, especially when it emanates from those we have generously helped or served wholeheartedly. This chapter tells the stories familiar to many – a tale of kindness-meeting-betrayal, trust-breaking, and the strength needed to rise above it.

The path to recovery is captured in a powerful quote by Maya Angelou, *"You may encounter many defeats, but you must not be defeated."* This sentiment echoes throughout the chapter, encouraging readers to find strength in their struggles and to view each challenge as an opportunity for growth. You are only defeated when you accept defeat.

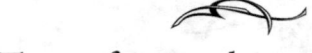

"The axe forgets; the tree remembers."
- African Proverb.

It does not matter how long you may have been hurt or criticised by the very people you try to help, I can tell you that it is possible to rise from the shadow of that hurt.

An African proverb says, *"The axe forgets; the tree remembers."* This poignant saying reminds us that while we may move on from acts of betrayal, the lessons we learn and the resilience we build form an integral part of our character. We may never truly forget the hurt meted on us by the very people we sought to help, but letting go by choosing the way of peace and love can usher us into dimensions of emotional healing we never thought possible.

The Cycle of Ungratefulness: A Personal Experience

In our journey through life, my husband and I have had the privilege of extending our hearts and hands to many around us, including friends, relatives, and some in our ministry.

This narrative tells the story of helping those who often saw our kindness not just as an act of love but something they were entitled to. It is a story that reflects not only the excessive kindness we have shown but also the tough lessons we have learned about ingratitude and the strength needed to keep a compassionate heart in a world that sometimes fails to value such virtues.

Among these friends, relatives, and ministry members, were several whose stories stood out, marked by a constant need and a lack of appreciation. We provided support in numerous ways — financial help during hard times, emotional support in challenging moments, and encouragement to help them find their path. However, our acts of love and care were often met with a sense of entitlement and no gratitude.

In all, we are often comforted with the principle in Genesis 8:22 — *"As long as the earth endures, seedtime and harvest, cold and heat, summer and winter, day and night will never cease."* The constant rhythm of sowing and reaping reminded us that every action has a reaction, deed, and consequence. This timeless truth helped us navigate the complexities of human behaviour, especially when our acts of kindness seemed to fall on barren ground. We realised that just as the earth undergoes cycles of planting and harvesting, so do our actions yield results, sometimes in ways we might not immediately see or understand.

This principle became particularly relevant as we dealt with individuals who took our generosity for granted. Each time we extended help, whether financial support during tough times, emotional backing in moments of distress, or encouragement to

"I've learnt that people will forget what you said, people will forget what you did, but people will never forget how you made them feel."
- Maya Angelou.

help them find their way, we were planting seeds. Initially, it was disheartening when these seeds appeared not to sprout — when our kindness was met with entitlement rather than gratitude.

One individual closely connected with us is particularly memorable in this cycle. Each instance of our assistance seemed only to deepen his expectation more. Our efforts to pull him out of financial troubles were seen not as gestures of love but as expected

>
> "The child who is not embraced by the village will burn it down to feel its warmth."
> - African Proverb.

duties. His habit of taking without giving and making promises he never kept slowly weakened the trust and affection we once had for him. The situation came to an end when he left, taking not just the financial aid we had offered but also a part of our trust and leaving behind a trail of broken promises that damaged our reputation.

Confronted with this disheartening reality, we found solace and direction in Proverbs

17:13, which states, *"Whoever rewards evil for good, evil will not depart from his house."* This verse became crucial to our belief system, reassuring us that justice and fairness will prevail, even if it is not in our hands to bring it about.

This journey, though filled with challenges, brought to mind an African proverb: *"The child who is not embraced by the village will burn it down to feel its warmth."* The saying highlights the tragic choices made by those who, feeling neglected or entitled, hurt those who have tried to help. Our experience reminded us of Maya Angelou's insightful words: *"I've learnt that people will forget what you said, people will forget what you did, but people will never forget how you made them feel."* This thought hit home for us, highlighting the lasting impact of our actions and intentions.

Permit me to share another ugly experience that stood out for my husband and me. My husband and I attended a church where we were actively involved as church workers. Despite our relentless dedication to assisting the Pastor of the church, we faced massive criticisms from within the church itself, especially from the family members of the Pastor.

>
> "Do not let what you cannot do interfere with what you can do."
> - Maya Angelou.

During this time, my husband encountered an attack on his character due to his loyalty and commitment to the Pastor. However, the situation took a more personal turn for me. I found myself not only physically attacked but also persecuted and heavily criticised for speaking out and defending my husband. This occurred when one of the Pastor's children verbally insulted him.

That event left me broken; nonetheless, we pressed forward in our commitment to the work of God. A few years later, fuelled by our faith and resilience, we started our ministry. The rest, they say, is history.

The lessons from the physical assaults, persecution, lack of gratitude, and criticisms became invaluable building blocks for where we find ourselves today. Those experiences, though challenging, served as a foundation for the strength and endurance required in ministry.

Ever since, God has been our Source of strength, guiding us through the trials and triumphs of our journey. The adversities we faced in the 1990s became stepping-stones, shaping our character and preparing us for the ministry we have today. The invaluable lessons from these unpleasant experiences became the bricks that helped us build a solid foundation for our future.

Before I share how these experiences helped shape us into who we have become today, let me share two significant reasons people feel entitled.

Why Do People Feel Entitled?

In this section, we explore the roots of ingratitude. Why do some individuals take kindness for granted? The answer lies in a mix of social conditioning, such as upbringing and belief.

Understanding these factors does not excuse their behaviour but helps us comprehend the complexities behind it.

Family Upbringing: A person's upbringing has much to do with how they approach life and respond to situations. The family is the child's first point of contact. As such, whatever they see around the home will likely form the foundation for their behaviour, beliefs, and approach to life.

For some, their upbringing did not encourage gratitude. For instance, a child who grew up not being appreciated may carry the attitude as they journey through life. There are families where members do not appreciate one another. In such a family setting, children hardly say 'thank you' to their parents in appreciation for their parental roles. They believe it is the parents' responsibility to do it, so they do not see it as a big deal.

>
> "The rain wets the leopard's spots but does not wash them off."
> - African Proverb.

Some parents, on the other hand, do not see the need to extend gratitude to their children when they run errands swiftly or do chores properly. Such parents feel it is the duty of the children. Hence, there is no need to thank them. This attitude can shape how children from that background will respond to the outside world.

Personal Beliefs: As people go through life, they form beliefs that become the basis for interacting with the world. Beliefs are so powerful and can determine many things in a person's life.

When people believe that being helped by others is something that is owed to them and that should be done for them, their response to acts of kindness will always be that of entitlement and ingratitude. Personal beliefs go a long way to determine how people respond to kindness and services rendered to them by other people.

Turning Pain into Lessons

Lessons from Life's Hard Knocks are vital in building one's future.

Life is an unpredictable journey. It often brings us face-to-face with challenges that test our patience, character, and understanding of human nature. This section gleans wisdom from real-life experiences, offering practical advice on navigating the complexities of human interactions, especially when faced with difficult people.

The most profound lessons often stem from the most challenging experiences. Here, we discuss how our ordeal taught us to set healthy boundaries, recognise potential exploitation, and prioritise self-care, even as we help others. Below are some of the lessons we have learned from our experiences.

Lesson One - How to Practice Kindness Sustainably

Our story, set in today's world where personal gain often seems more essential than community well-being, is a stark reminder of the enduring power of compassion. Despite these experiences, we have learnt to remain dedicated to helping others. Now, we do it with a wisdom that ensures our generosity and considers our well-being. This journey has taught us the vital balance between giving and self-care, ensuring that our future acts of kindness are as much a gift to ourselves as they are to others. In a nutshell, *"You cannot pour from an empty cup,"* which implies taking care of oneself is essential to taking care of others effectively. The idea is to practice kindness and generosity in a sustainable way that allows for your well-being and longevity in being able to help others. Therefore, do good but let your kindness be in moderation.

Lesson Two - How to Manage Expectations When Helping Others

When we extend help to others, it is natural to hope for appreciation or positive outcomes. However, managing our expectations is crucial. A powerful quote by John Wooden aptly states, *"Do not let what you cannot do interfere with what you can do."* This reminds us to focus on our ability to offer help instead of becoming entangled in expectations about the results or recognition of our actions. Our experiences with these folks taught us how to manage expectations while helping people.

Lesson Three - Understanding the Hard Truths about Human Nature

Human nature is complex and often contradictory. It is a blend of good and bad, gratefulness and ingratitude. An African proverb says, *"The rain wets the leopard's spots but does not wash them off."* Similarly, our experiences with people might change our perceptions but should not alter our core values and beliefs. We must learn to accept the reality of human imperfection while maintaining our integrity and kindness.

Lesson Four - How to Deal with Difficult People

Interacting with difficult individuals is inevitable. It is important to remember that we cannot control others' actions, but we can control our reactions. The Bible offers guidance in Proverbs 15:1, *"A gentle answer turns away wrath, but a harsh word stirs up anger."* This verse reminds us of the power of calmness and kindness in the face of provocation. Responding with patience and understanding can often diffuse tension and lead to more positive outcomes.

Lesson Five – How to Set Healthy Boundaries

Learning to set healthy boundaries is a great way to help others while denying them an opportunity to hurt you. In our case, this lesson becomes necessary to protect ourselves while extending generosity to people.

The Power of Letting Go

Forgiveness is not about condoning wrongdoings but freeing ourselves from resentment. This part of the chapter delves into the process of letting go. It is a journey that is often difficult but ultimately liberating, allowing us to move on from the hurt while retaining the lessons learnt.

Through this process, I truly came to terms with the fact that forgiveness is freedom. Letting go allows you to heal and forge ahead in life.

Unforgiveness and resentment can hinder you from making headways if left unattended. This is why letting go is first a gift to yourself rather than the offender. While letting go may not wipe out the memory of what happened, it will bring you the liberty and healing you need to progress.

EMBRACE EVERY MOMENT

Walk away from the people and things that consistently hurt you, but ensure not to carry the needless burden of unforgiveness as you do so. Walking away is vital, but forgiving is even more vital.

Finally, it is important to learn from any negative experiences you may have had. Embrace the lessons that life has taught you, and use them to grow and create a better future for yourself. Every moment in life is an opportunity to learn and improve, even the difficult ones. So please make the most of them and keep striving towards your goals.

www.ingramcontent.com/pod-product-compliance
Lightning Source LLC
Chambersburg PA
CBHW070406120526
44590CB00014B/1275